GASTROINTESTINAL PATHOLOGY

Dr. Kavita Ramanathan

ALLIED HEALTH PRESS

Gastrointestinal Pathology

Author: **Dr. Kavita Ramanathan**

Allied Health Press
4164 Lakeshore Road
Burlington ON L7L 1A4
Canada
www.alliedhealthpress.com
Email: orders@arclereducation.com

ISBN: 978-1-77956-764-2

ABOUT THE AUTHOR

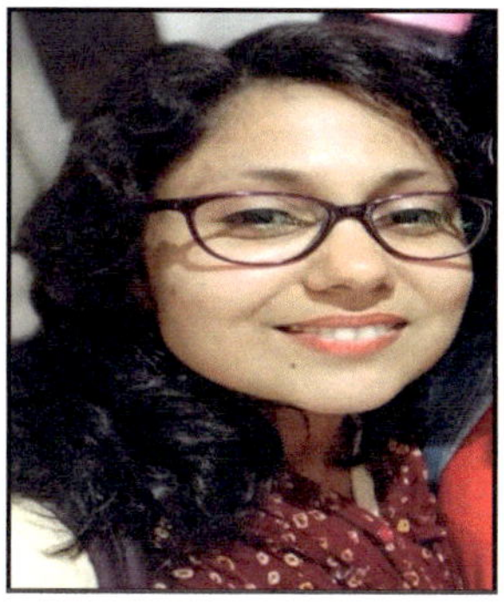

Dr Kavita Ramanathan is an accomplished medical professional with experience working through the length and breadth of India. With 16+ years in clinical and anatomic pathology, she understands the normal and abnormal functioning of the human body in depth. Also, she held positions in the senior management for 8+ years and designed business strategies. She successfully helped organisations attain profitability while maintaining quality and service standards. Additionally, during the COVID-19 pandemic, she contributed significantly by aligning operations to support government initiatives. She earned her undergraduate and graduate medical degrees from reputed institutions under the University of Mumbai, India, and she also holds an MBA in Finance. Dr Kavita volunteers with a non-profit organisation where she tutors students from low-income schools for over two decades. Post-pandemic, she quit her corporate job to pursue her passion of teaching and writing. Currently, she tutors high school and university students in biology, psychology, and medical sciences. Additionally, she authors books, articles, and blogs on topics related to health and well-being. Her strong academic background, enriched with a vast and varied experience, shapes her into a mature and sensible professional.

Brief Table of Contents

Detailed Table of Contents

CHAPTER 4

Bioactive Foods and Chronic GI Diseases 51

CHAPTER 5

GI Diseases and Dietary Interventions 67

CHAPTER 6

Molecular Pathology of GI Diseases 83

CHAPTER 7

Drug Therapy for GI Diseases 95

LIST OF FIGURES

PREFACE

Despite having different pathologies and spatial distributions, colorectal cancer (CRC) and peptic ulcer disease (PUD) have a significant global impact. An estimated 1.4 million cases of CRC and around 90 million new cases of PUD are reported annually. For both conditions, early diagnosis and treatment are essential for successful management, but their availability is limited and costs are high. Furthermore, PUD and CRC are nearly unavoidable due to the widespread presence of *Helicobacter pylori* (the primary cause of PUD) and societal and environmental factors that strongly influence disease development. However, it is thought that promoting a healthy lifestyle and increasing knowledge of the epidemiology of PUD and CRC, along with the factors underlying their etiopathology, can help reduce cases.

Over the decades, several factors have revolutionized the treatment of gastrointestinal diseases. When cimetidine, an H2 receptor antagonist and the first powerful acid-inhibitory medication, became available in 1976, it was believed that reflux and peptic ulcer disease would be eradicated. Proton pump inhibitors, which were even more effective, soon followed. The identification of *Helicobacter pylori* and the development of triple therapy marked another significant advancement in ulcer disease management. The bioactive amine 5-hydroxytryptamine (5-HT) plays a crucial role in gastrointestinal function, leading to the development of various antagonists with significant therapeutic potential. For example, 5-HT3 receptor antagonists are important for reducing chemotherapy-induced nausea and may also be useful in treating functional issues such as irritable bowel syndrome (IBS).

Future research must address several issues, such as developing more potent drugs to alter gastrointestinal motility, reducing damage caused by acute pancreatitis, and creating therapeutically effective medications for managing gastric diseases.

This book provides an introduction to gastrointestinal diseases (GIDs) with relevant examples and is a valuable resource for students interested in understanding GIDs and their treatments.

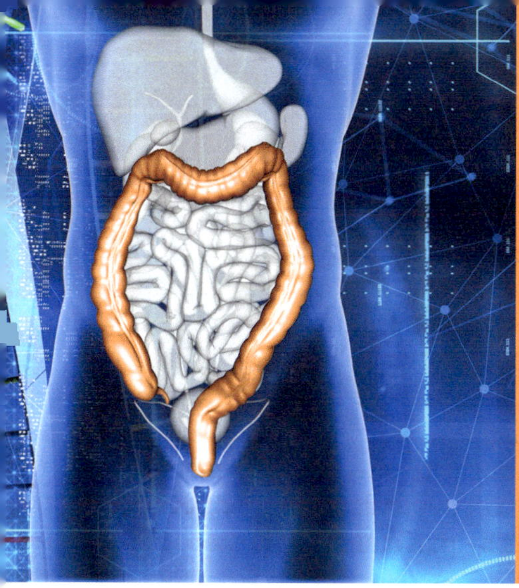

Chapter 1

INTRODUCTION TO GASTROINTESTINAL PATHOLOGY

Contents

1.1. Introduction

The diaphragm, pancreas, and transverse mesocolon are among the organs that make up the visceral bed on which the muscular, J-shaped stomach rests (Ban, 2024). The quantity of food within the stomach, the stage of digestion at which it is, the degree of development of the gastric muscles, and the state of the surrounding intestines all affect how the stomach interacts with the surrounding viscera. The empty stomach is only a little larger than a fist, yet it has the capacity to store up to 4 L of food and liquid before contracting back to its resting size (Daniels and Allum, 2005). The duodenum and the esophagus are joined to the stomach at the gastroesophageal junction (Figure 1.1).

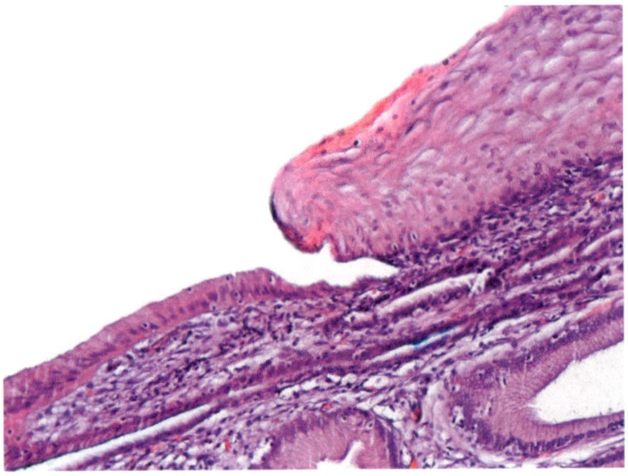

Figure 1.1. *Gastroesophageal junction.*

Source: https://upload.wikimedia.org/wikipedia/commons/c/c5/Gastroesophageal_junction%2C_high_mag.jpg, Creative Commons License.

1.2. Stomach

The stomach can be separated into five sections based on histological differences, such as "cardia" (located below the esophagus) has a cardiac sphincter that keeps stomach contents from reentering the esophagus. The "fundus" (located below the diaphragm) and to the left of the cardia, typically contains air and can be seen on radiographs.

The "body" is the portion of the stomach that is used for breaking down (digesting) food. The partially digested food will be waiting to be released into the small intestine in the "pyloric antrum." The "pyloric canal," which is found in this area, regulates the flow of food that has been digested from the stomach to the duodenum and keeps its contents from returning to the stomach. The pyloric canal attaches the stomach to the small intestine. When food is not present, the stomach contracts inward, causing the mucosa and submucosa to form a fold known as a ruga. The stomach wall is made up of multiple layers. The mucosa or the mucous membrane is the inner lining and is made up of three parts: the muscularis mucosae, the lamina propria, and the epithelial lining. The stomach lining is protected by specialized cells called parietal cells, which produce hydrochloric acid, chief cells, which produce the proteolytic enzyme pepsin, mucous cells, or goblet cells, which make up the surface layer of the simple columnar epithelium, and hormones, such as gastrin. The ability of the small intestine to absorb vitamin B_{12} depends on the secretion of intrinsic factors by parietal cells (Festen, 1991) (Figure 1.2).

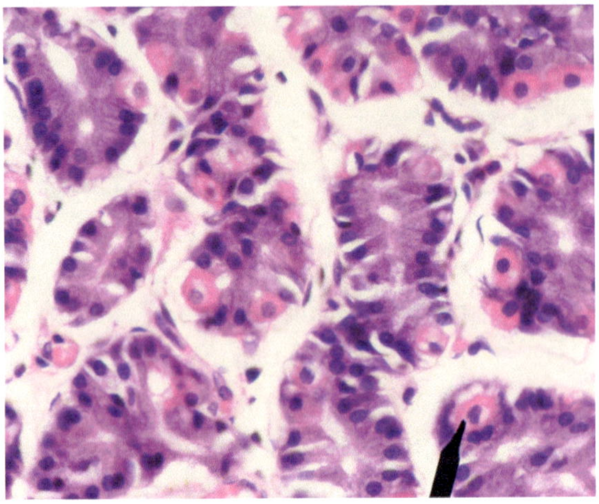

Figure 1.2. *Parietal cells.*

Source: https://upload.wikimedia.org/wikipedia/commons/5/5a/Parietal_cells.jpg, Creative Commons License.

The submucosa is a layer of loose areolar tissue that has some elastic fibers and is made up of nerve cells, blood vessels, and lymph vessels. The primary layer of smooth muscles in the wall is called the muscularis propria or muscularis externa. It is composed of three layers: an inner oblique layer, a middle circular layer, and an outer longitudinal layer. The serosa or visceral peritoneum, is the thin outer layer of loose connective tissue that covers the stomach. Hormonal and neural impulses govern the motility and secretion of the stomach. The stomach is innervated from multiple directions. Parasympathetic fibers travel in the gastric branches of the vagi. The sensory vagal fibers include fibers related with secretion (gastric). The sympathetic fibers supply blood vessels and musculature via the splanchnic nerves and celiac ganglia. Many hormones have been shown to affect stomach motility; for instance, cholecystokinin, and gastrin relax the proximal stomach and increase distal stomach contractions. There are three stages to stomach secretion. They are intestinal, gastric, and cephalic secretions.

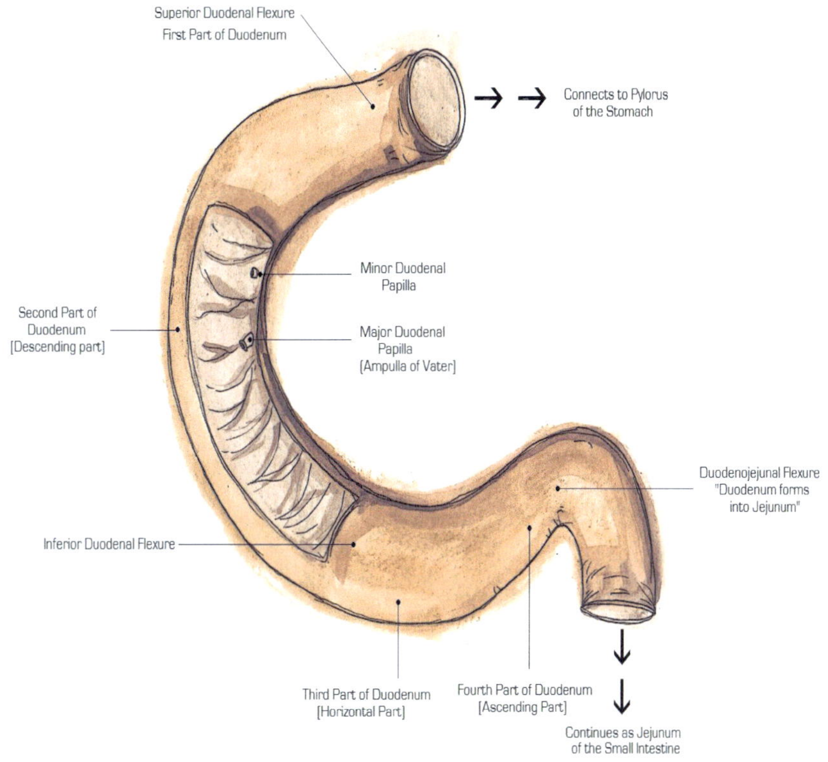

Figure 1.3. *Duodenum.*

Source: https://upload.wikimedia.org/wikipedia/commons/3/35/Duodenumanatomy.jpg, Creative Commons License.

The food passes through the relatively short cephalic phase (reflex phase) of gastric secretion before entering the stomach. This stage is triggered by the smell, taste, sight, and gastric secretion is now a conditioned reflex. The introduction of food into the stomach stimulates local neural and hormonal systems, which cause the 3-to-4-hour gastric phase of secretion (Spainhour, 2018). There are both excitatory and inhibitory components in the intestinal phase of gastric secretion. During this stage, the duodenum plays a significant role in controlling the stomach emptying phase. Food is mixed and digested in the stomach, which also serves as a temporary storage space for food. Food in the stomach turns into a liquid known as chyme, which is discharged into the duodenum for absorption through periodic contractions of the pyloric section of the muscles. During the gastric emptying process, the pyloric sphincter is forced to open and allow roughly 3 ml of chyme to pass through at a time into the duodenum by repetitive mixing waves. The remaining chyme is forced back into the stomach, where it continues to mix. When more chyme is forced into the duodenum by the subsequent mixing waves, this process is repeated. While water, alcohol, and other lipid-soluble substances, such as aspirin and other NSAIDs, may move from the stomach into the circulation, the stomach does not permit substantial food absorption. The ileum often empties into the large intestine upon food entry into the stomach and this is called gastroileal reflex (Costa and Furness, 1982). The duodenum is a C-shaped organ that connects the duodenojejunal flexure to the pylorus. It is divided into four anatomical sections. The bile, pancreatic, and accessory pancreatic ducts enter the second half of the duodenum, and each duct is normally protected by a sphincter. The pancreatic and bile ducts will join to form a hepatopancreatic ampulla. The duodenum performs similar functions to other regions of the small intestine, such as chemical and mechanical digestion and nutritional absorption. Within 2–4 hours of the meal, the stomach contents are entirely evacuated into the duodenum (Figure 1.3). The food materials that are high in protein take longer to digest than materials that are high in carbohydrates, which empty the stomach first. When the duodenum is processing fatty chyme, food can stay in the stomach for up to six hours because small intestine enzymes break down fats slowly (Wahlqvist and Wattanapenpaiboon, 2020).

1.3. Mucosa

In order for our food to be properly digested, the stomach is essential. This organ is resistant to a wide range of harmful substances, such as alcohol, hydrochloric acid (HCL), refluxed bile salts, and other irritants (agents). Numerous physiological defensive mechanisms and the capacity for quick mucosal healing in the event of injury allow the body to maintain this high resistance to damage. However, a stomach mucosal lesion (gastric erosion) and ulcer may arise when these defense systems are overpowered by irritating stimuli. The mucosal barrier is altered by aggressive factors, which leads to damage to the epithelial cells. In the peptic ulcer disease (PUD), the roles of a number of variables, including pepsin, gastric acid, and *Helicobacter pylori* (*H. pylori*), are now well documented (Chan and Leung, 2002). It is commonly known that the *H. pylori* infection, gastric acid, and pepsin play a vital role in the development of PUD.

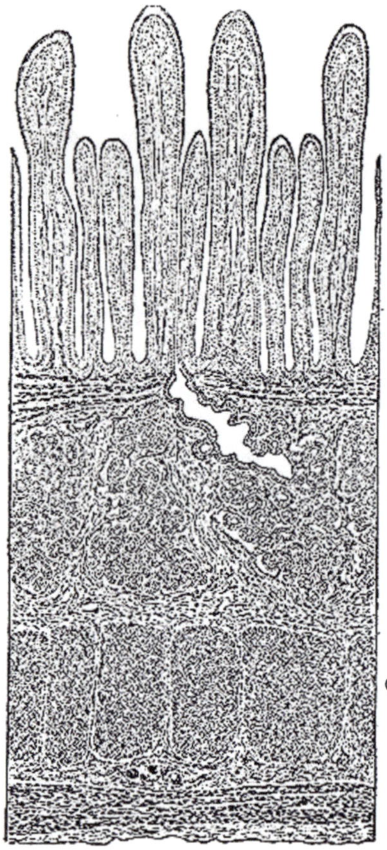

Figure 1.4. *Muscularis mucosa.*

Source: https://upload.wikimedia.org/wikipedia/commons/5/54/Gray1058.png, Creative Commons License.

However, new research indicates that other variables, including obesity and smoking, may also play a vital role in the onset of peptic ulcer disease and may even be risk factors for the disease progression. The stomach and duodenal mucosal defense systems and gastric acid secretion are in a state of physiological balance under normal conditions. When this delicate balance is upset, mucosal damage occurs. Peptic ulcers are therefore described as abnormalities in the submucosa and mucosa of the stomach or duodenum that penetrate the muscularis mucosa (Figure 1.4). When the stomach and duodenum epithelial cells are stimulated by cholinergic substances or when their lining becomes irritated, they release mucus. Mucus and bicarbonate, which are produced by the foveolar cells, combine to create a gel layer that is impervious to aggressive substances like acid and pepsin. Because it keeps the stomach from digesting itself, this layer is crucial. Other processes aid in preventing pepsin and acid from penetrating the damaged epithelium cells. Improved blood flow eliminates (removes) acid that permeates the injured mucosa and gives epithelial cells in the gel layer a sufficient bicarbonate level at the surface. Through the ion pumps in the basolateral cell membrane, epithelial cells eliminate excess hydrogen ions to control the pH of the intracellular environment. When the equilibrium between aggressive agents and the defense mechanism is upset, mucosal damage and, consequently, peptic ulcers, arise. *H. pylori* infection, NSAIDs, alcohol, bile salts, acid, and pepsin are examples of aggressive factors. Mucus, bicarbonate, prostaglandins, sufficient mucosal blood flow, and the capacity for epithelium regeneration are all components of the defense system. The bicarbonate barrier and mucus provide the initial (first) line of defense for the stomach mucosa. Bicarbonate anions and mucus gel combine to form a layer that covers the surface of the gastric mucosa (Allen and Flemström, 2005). The layer can hold on to the bicarbonate ions released by surface epithelial cells and keep the pH close to 7 when it comes to the mucosa. The mucous layer can also shield the epithelium from pepsin proteolytic effects. Almost 95% of the mucus gel that foveolar cells make is made up of water and several mucin glycoproteins, including MUC2, MUC5AC, MUC6, etc (Taherali et al., 2018). The capacity of mucin units to polymerize into extended (large) mucin multimers makes gel formation feasible. The regulation of gastric mucus secretion is influenced by several GI hormones, including prostaglandins, secretin, and gastrin. The first line of defense against gastric acid is the pH gradient that is maintained at the epithelial surface due to the release of bicarbonate into the mucus gel layer. Surface epithelial cells release bicarbonate anions from their apical membrane. Many substances, including prostaglandins, luminal acid, orexin-A, and melatonin can stimulate the Cl^-/HCO_3^- exchanger, which controls the secretion of bicarbonate (Sjöblom, 2005).

1.4. Protective Mechanisms

The only mechanism that divides the lumen from the epithelium is the mucus-bicarbonate barrier. Other protective mechanisms are therefore triggered when the barrier to protection breaks down due to pathological events or when injuring (irritants) agents exert their influence. They consist of mucosal blood flow maintenance, fast epithelial tissue renewal, and intracellular acid neutralization. Prostaglandins, particularly PGE2 and PGI2, are continuously produced by the gastric mucosa and are essential for maintaining mucosal integrity and shielding it from harmful substances (Seddighi and Lee, 2016). Prostaglandins have been shown to interact with nearly every mucosal defense mechanism. Specifically, they may lessen the generation of acid, promote the creation of mucus and bicarbonate, and improve blood flow to the mucosa. It is also because prostaglandins speed up mucosal healing and epithelial restoration. Moreover, prostaglandins can prevent leukocyte adherence to vascular endothelium and mast cell activation. The next line of mucosal defense is made up of a continuous layer of surface epithelial cells joined by tight junctions. Tight connections enable epithelial cells to establish an impermeable barrier that stops pepsin and gastric acid from invading the stomach and causing damage to the deeper layers. Because they have phospholipids on their surface, epithelial cells are hydrophobic and can repel substances that dissolve in water and acid and cause harm to mucous membranes. Cathelicidins and beta-defensins are produced by epithelial cells. These cationic peptides protect against bacterial colonization of the stomach mucosa and are crucial to the innate defensive mechanism at the mucosal surface. Mucosal progenitor cells continuously renew their cells, preserving the integrity of the continuous layer of surface epithelial cells. While the entire process of epithelial renewal takes three to seven days, the restoration of epithelium following exposure to harmful chemicals happens in a matter of minutes and is dependent on the migration of preserved cells from the gastric glands. Growth factors like insulin-like growth factor 1 or IGF-1 and transforming growth factor-α or TGF-α, regulate the proliferation of progenitor cells. The primary growth factor receptor in gastric progenitor cells is the epidermal growth factor receptor or EGFR, which is activated by several growth factors. Gastrin and prostaglandins (PGE_2) interact with EGFR to promote gastric mucosal cell renewal and proliferation (Yan et al., 2009). The gastric mucosa does not expressed EGF on its own. However, it is produced by the salivary and esophageal glands and is present in the stomach lumen. In the event of an injury, it can promote the proliferation of progenitor cells.

1.5. Blood Flow Dynamics

Ensuring sufficient blood flow to the mucosa is essential for the delivery of essential chemicals, including oxygen and nutrients, as well as the elimination of harmful compounds from the mucosa. Potent vasodilators like prostacyclin and nitric oxide (NO), which are produced by endothelial cells found in the capillaries, shield the gastric mucosa from the damaging effects of reduced blood flow (Abdel-Sala et al., 2001). Following exposure to irritants, the mucosal blood flow increases quickly. This procedure makes it possible to dilute stomach acid and remove harmful substances. A reduction in blood flow leads to the development of tissue necrosis, and adequate blood flow is essential for preventing injury to the gastric mucosa. Experimental data demonstrate that NO mediates the increase in mucosal blood flow and that blocking NO synthase worsens mucosal damage. The urease-producing ability of the gram-negative *H. pylori* is one of its adaptation traits that help it thrive in the acidic, unfavorable environment, where it causes inflammation and produces peptic ulcer disease. *H. pylori* first colonizes the antrum, which lacks parietal cells, which secrete gastric acid, so acid secretion is not immediately impacted. In general, there are several steps involved in the mechanism by which these bacteria cause disease. The bacteria first penetrate the mucous layer of the stomach, interfere with the antimicrobial action of the gastric acid barrier, and adjust to the environmental conditions of the mucus. The second stage involves *H. pylori* adhering to the gastric mucosa. This causes the production of multiple bacterial genes, enabling the pathogen to survive in this environment and evade certain actions brought on by peristaltic motions or mucous layer shedding. The urease enzyme, which can convert urea into ammonia and carbon dioxide to raise the pH to neutral by creating an acid-neutralizing cloud of ammonia close to the bacterium and shielding it from stomach acid, is one of the key components in *H. pylori* colonization.

1.6. Inflammation

Inflammatory cells such as polymorphonuclear leukocytes, lymphocytes, plasma cells, and macrophages infiltrate the stomach mucosa in *H. pylori* gastritis (Figure 1.5) (Crabtree, 1996). *H. pylori* produce lipase and protease, which break down gastric mucus and cause damage to cells when gastric acid is reintroduced. Ammonia generated by urease action could be harmful to the cells that line the stomach. *H. pylori* infection causes the stomach mucosa to experience chronic oxidative stress, which damages the mucosa and slows down the process of mucosal repair. The stomach secretes a fluid called gastric acid, which stimulates digestive enzymes and assists in the breakdown of proteins. Hydrochloric acid (HCL), which is produced by parietal cells in the gastric gland, is the primary component of gastric acid. The stomach lumen has a pH between 1.5 and 3.5 due to gastric acid. The process of controlling stomach acid output involves four different cell types: enterochromaffin-like cells, parietal cells, D cells, and G cells. The autonomic nervous system and hormones, including histamine, cholecystokinin, vasoactive intestinal peptide, and others, also control the generation of gastric acid. Gastric acid output is significantly impacted by *H. pylori* infection. Patients with *H. pylori* infections likely produce less acid than usual because pro-inflammatory mediators cause apoptosis. *H. pylori* infection could result in more acid being secreted. Gastrin, an acid-stimulating hormone, is released more frequently when there is an *H. pylori* infection (Kaneko et al., 2002). Prolonged hypergastrinemia leads to the growth of parietal cells and increased acid production, which can lead to the growth of ulcers, particularly in the duodenum. Increased duodenal acid load brought on by elevated gastric acid output harms the mucosa and results in ulcers. The proenzyme pepsinogen, the precursor to pepsin, is synthesized and released by the chief cells. They are present in the body, fundus, and antrum, and many cells in the gastric mucosa. The main digesting protease in the gastric juice is pepsin, a member of the peptidase A1 family. Pepsin damage differs significantly from that caused by ethanol or NaCl, which quickly cross the mucus barrier and cause the epithelial layer to exfoliate, increasing mucosal permeability. Reepithelialization then occurs beneath a fibrin-based mucoid cap.

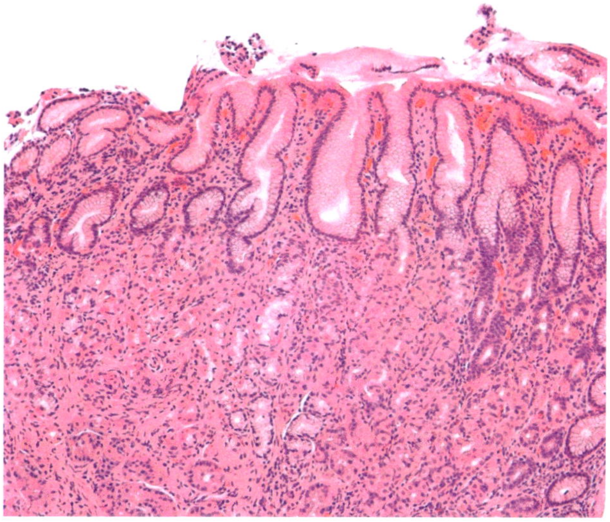

Figure 1.5. *H. pylori gastritis.*

Source: https://upload.wikimedia.org/wikipedia/commons/5/58/Gastritis_helicobacter_-_intermed_mag.jpg, Creative Commons License.

1.7. Biochemistry of Drugs

Luminal pepsin cannot penetrate the adhering mucus gel layer, preventing it from reaching the underlying mucosa. Pepsin is unable to penetrate the continuous mucus layer within a short time due to its large molecular size. The mucus layer is gradually hydrolyzed and eroded by luminal pepsin at an acidic pH. Further research is needed to fully understand the relationship between pepsin-induced mucosal injury and PUD. The preference of PUD patients for acid-inhibiting drugs over pepsin as a mucosal-damaging agent may account for this lack of interest in the digestive enzyme. It was believed that the majority of the pepsin activity *in vivo* is lost beyond pH 3, as the proteolytic activity of pepsin in gastric juice rapidly decreases above this pH. Arachidonic acid is converted to prostaglandins when prostaglandin synthases and cyclooxygenases (COX-1 and COX-2) are present (Morita, 2002). Because NSAIDs inhibit cyclooxygenases, there is a strong correlation between the inhibition of prostaglandin production and gastrointestinal damage caused by their ingestion. Many prostaglandin-related protective actions are suppressed when cyclooxygenases are inhibited. For example, prostaglandins suppress leukocyte adherence to vascular endothelium and decrease mast cell activation. Prostaglandins also help to keep mucosal microcirculation blood flow at a sufficient level. When NSAIDs are administered, bicarbonate secretion is inhibited (cyclooxygenase-dependent), which also comprises the mucosal defense system. One cause of PUD is nonsteroidal anti-inflammatory medication. Up to 25% of individuals who regularly take NSAIDs report having an ulcer, up to 50% report gastrointestinal intolerance, and up to 5% experience gastrointestinal complications (Peura, 2004). These medications affect the mucosa in both cyclooxygenase-dependent and cyclooxygenase-independent ways by breaking down the mucosal permeability barrier. Patients who use NSAIDs on a regular basis have a reduction in stomach and duodenal ulcerations as well as complications from these conditions, although not a complete elimination. A low dose of aspirin used to prevent cardiovascular disease (CVD) was linked to a higher risk of ulcer and complications.

Almost 90% of gastric and duodenal ulcers (Figure 1.6) are caused by *H. pylori* infection and NSAIDs (Venerito and Malfertheiner, 2010). Therefore, understanding the role that NSAIDs and *H. pylori* infection play in the pathophysiology of PUD is crucial for both ulcer treatment and prevention. NSAIDs and *H. pylori* may have additive or synergistic negative effects on the mucosa. Though the connection between *H. pylori* infections and NSAIDs is biologically known, but there is ongoing debate regarding the combined causal roles of those risk factors in ulcer formation. While some studies failed to find a connection between the presence of *H. pylori* infection and an increase in NSAID-associated damage, others did. However, recent studies revealed that *H. pylori*-infected individuals in Denmark had an almost twofold increased risk of bleeding from a peptic ulcer compared to those who were not infected. Some researchers suggest that NSAID use increased the incidence of peptic ulcers by three and five times, respectively, in individuals with and without *H. pylori*. Research on the genetic background as a potential risk factor for PUD dates back to a period before *H. pylori* was discovered and linked to peptic ulcers. These investigations revealed that PUD may be caused by a polygenic inheritance pattern. There is a threefold rise in the prevalence of gastric ulcers but no duodenal ulcers among first-degree relatives of individuals with gastric ulcers. However, there is a three-fold increase in the frequency of duodenal ulcers but no gastric ulcers in first-degree relatives of patients with duodenal ulcers.

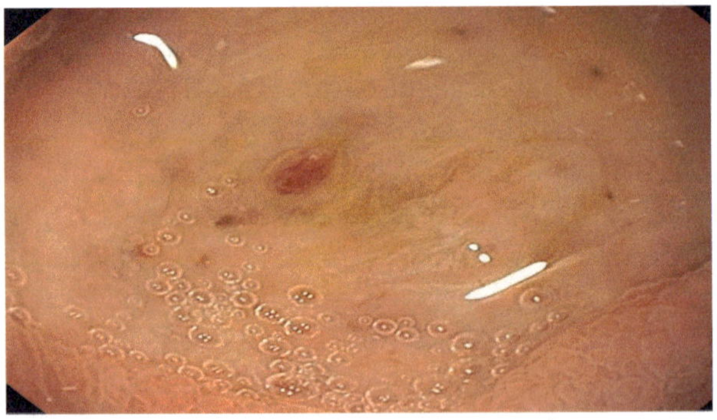

Figure 1.6. *Duodenal ulcer.*

Source: https://upload.wikimedia.org/wikipedia/commons/3/3e/Duodenal_ulcer.jpg, Creative Commons License.

1.8. Gastrointestinal Disorders

Gastrointestinal disorders like acid reflux, gallstones (Figure 1.7), and cancers of the colon, esophagus, and pancreas are linked to obesity (Camilleri et al., 2017). Patients who are obese have an excess of visceral adipose tissue. It is known that visceral adipose tissue is active and has been linked to higher concentrations of cytokines that promote inflammation in the gastrointestinal tract. Therefore, it has been suggested that obesity may have an impact on PUD. Some researchers discovered that obesity is a risk factor for gastric ulcers but not duodenal ulcers. However, no difference in stomach ulcer and duodenal ulcer was detected between obese and non-obese patients. Thus, there is ongoing debate over a potential link between obesity and PUD. There was no difference in the incidence of *H. pylori* infection between obese patients and non-obese persons, indicating that obesity rather than *H. pylori* is responsible for the higher prevalence of gastritis.

The largest avoidable risk factor for human disease is smoking. Smoking cigarettes has been linked to lung conditions, malignancies, and cardiovascular diseases. Smoking causes health problems for people and is therefore a major public health concern. Cigarette smoke contains about 5000 different chemicals, at least 150 of which are known to be harmful or carcinogenic (Baker, 2006). Alkaloids, phenolic chemicals, nitrosamines, polycyclic aromatic hydrocarbons, and heavy metals are some of these components. All of these substances can worsen lipid peroxidation, which is the precursor to atherosclerosis, and cause oxidative stress in smokers. Significantly, smoking causes 70% of non-small cell lung cancer cases and 90% of small cell lung cancer cases globally (Gridelli et al., 2015). These days, there is ample evidence linking cigarette smoking to gastrointestinal diseases, among which chronic inflammation is a major contributing factor. These comprise GI tract malignancies, inflammatory bowel disease, and peptic ulcers.

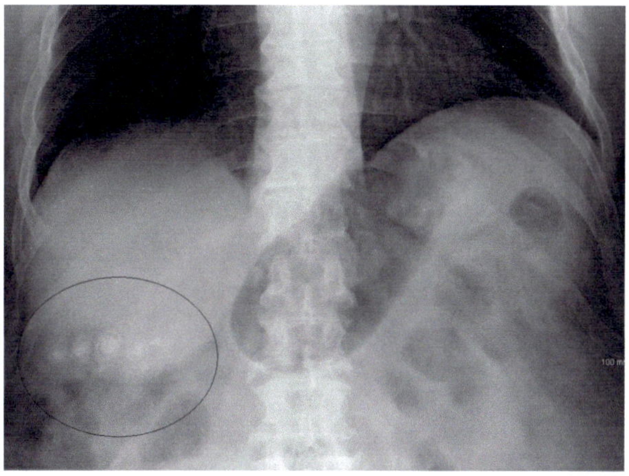

Figure 1.7. *Gallstones.*

Source: https://upload.wikimedia.org/wikipedia/commons/d/de/StonesXray.PNG, Creative Commons License.

Smokers who use large amounts of tobacco on a daily basis are more likely to develop peptic ulcers. Smoking alters the stomach mucosal protective system, raising the chance of *H. pylori* infection, but it is not an independent ulcerogenic agent. Alcohol consumption and ulcers can be associated. Alcohol use, whether acute or chronic, can affect stomach function in a number of ways. For example, alcohol can cause acute stomach mucosal damage and change the secretion of gastric acid. While alcoholic beverages with a higher alcohol level do not promote either gastric acid secretion or gastric release, those with a lower alcohol content increase both. Several investigations have revealed a connection between alcohol-induced mucosal damage and a reduction in prostaglandin synthesis. It is often documented that drinking alcohol can inflame the mucosa, which can harm the mucosa. Alcohol increases the permeability of the mucosa and damages the stomach mucosal barrier. The alterations brought about by brief exposure to alcohol can be quickly reversed, however, continuous alcohol consumption might cause microcirculation problems and worsen structural mucosal damage. Alcohol usage in the past was linked to a higher likelihood of having an ulcer history. One of the popular drinks consumed worldwide is coffee. GERD, or gastroesophageal reflux disease, (Figure 1.8), and peptic ulcer disease have been linked to coffee use (Locke et al., 1999). While there is no conclusive evidence linking caffeine to the pathophysiology of peptic ulcer disease, it is typically advised to avoid coffee drinks.

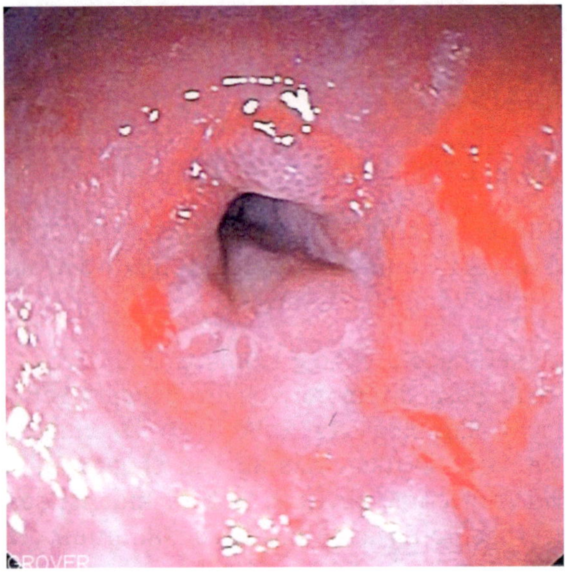

Figure 1.8. *Gastroesophageal reflux disease.*

Source: https://upload.wikimedia.org/wikipedia/commons/1/16/Peptic_stricture.png, Creative Commons License.

Because of its phosphodiesterase inhibitory action and ability to increase cyclic AMP, caffeine is thought to enhance the release of gastric acid. Some researchers have shown that drinking decaffeinated coffee increases the production of gastric acid. Decaffeinated and normal coffee are more effective stimulants of gastric acid release than caffeine alone (Liszt et al., 2017). Once the symptoms of peptic ulcer disease appeared, patients with duodenal ulcers either decreased the amount of coffee they consumed or quit altogether. Some studies indicate a strong relationship between the quantity of coffee consumed by patients with duodenal ulcers and the symptoms that mimic ulcers. However, a lot of research studies indicate that there is no connection between coffee consumption and peptic ulcer disease.

1.9. Discomfort

Identifying PUD at an early stage can be challenging. Before major complications like gastrointestinal bleeding occur, peptic ulcers may show up as dyspeptic or other gastrointestinal symptoms, or they may show no symptoms at all. PUD symptoms are not sensitive or specific enough to provide an accurate diagnosis. Therefore, more testing is required to verify the diagnosis and start the proper course of treatment. Abdominal pain, bloating, and fullness are clinical manifestations we can observe. There may also be weight loss, nausea, and vomiting. For patients with PUD, upper abdomen pain or discomfort is the most common symptom. Epigastric discomfort affects about 80% of people with PUD who obtain an endoscopic diagnosis (Lu et al., 2004). Even while pain or discomfort is frequently concentrated in the epigastrium, it can also happen in the upper quadrants on the right or left. Atypical and extremely rare is the major symptom of pain radiating to the back. The timing of the symptoms in relation to the food consumed may aid in characterizing duodenal ulcers from gastric ulcers. Duodenal ulcer symptoms appear 2–4 hours after a meal when the stomach begins to leak digested food and gastric acid into the duodenum. In contrast, symptoms of a gastric ulcer would cause epigastric pain during or immediately after the meal due to increased gastric acid production. The pain linked to duodenal ulcers happens when there is no food, since food buffers the acid in the stomach.

1.10. Other Aspects

The peak period for circadian acid stimulation (11 PM and 2 AM) is when discomfort related to duodenal ulcers develops. The effects of food, alkali, and antisecretory medications like proton pump inhibitors or H2-receptor antagonists imply that gastric acid is a major factor in the development of symptoms. People without duodenal ulcers did not experience discomfort when hydrochloric acid was infused into the duodenum. Giant ulcers are often more than 2 cm in diameter and might exhibit back pain that radiates. Individuals with giant ulcers may experience weight loss even in the absence of cancer. They can become more complicated due to pyloric obstruction, posterior penetration, or bleeding. Many risk factors, including age, *H. pylori* infection, NSAID use, methamphetamine, or cocaine use, have been linked to the development of giant ulcers. Comorbidities appear to be a major factor in the development of these ulcers; they have been linked to lung transplantation, end-stage renal failure, and Crohn's disease. Pyloric channel ulcers are often accompanied by pain that starts soon after eating and vomiting. Pyloric dysfunction or blockage can cause vomiting. Postbulbar ulcers are usually seen 1–3 cm from the pylorus in the duodenal bulb (Yaghoobi and Armstrong, 2022). There is no specific clinical characteristic that helps differentiate postbulbar ulcers from other types of ulcers. However, this type of ulcer has been documented to have a high prevalence of complications. Postbulbar ulcers may cause gastrinoma.

Food consumption can cause early satiety, fatty food intolerance, nausea, or sporadic vomiting, as well as epigastric fullness, postprandial belching, and epigastric pain that gets worse with eating. The changes in visceral sensitization and gastroduodenal motility appear to be linked to food-initiated symptoms in PUD patients. Dyspepsia or other gastrointestinal symptoms were absent in 43–87% of patients with bleeding peptic ulcers (Barkun and Leontiadis, 2010). Moreover, perforations in the stomach ulcer may occur without any prior symptoms. Patients who are old or who may be on NSAIDs may be asymptomatic. Those who have an asymptomatic ulcer are more likely to experience major PUD complications like bleeding or perforation. Ulcers may be revealed during an endoscopic examination of these asymptomatic people. PUD complications have led to fewer hospitalizations recently, along with a decline in PUD prevalence. However, if PUD is left untreated, it may worsen due to potentially fatal complications from ulcers, including gastrointestinal bleeding, perforation, and gastric outlet obstruction (GOO) (Figure 1.9).

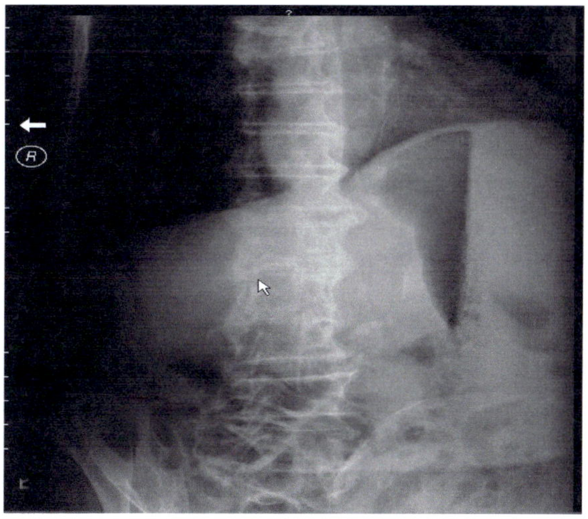

Figure 1.9. *Gastric outlet obstruction.*

Source: https://upload.wikimedia.org/wikipedia/commons/5/5b/GOO_AXR.jpg, Creative Commons License.

It is crucial to keep in mind that complications in patients with PUD can arise from any cause; yet, it is evident that *H. pylori* infections and NSAID use are the main contributors to ulcer bleeding and perforation. New ulcer symptoms, a change in symptoms, or an unexpected occurrence in the absence of normal symptoms can all be signs of complications. One prevalent problem that leads to high morbidity and medical care expenditures is upper gastrointestinal hemorrhage caused by PUD. The two main signs are melena and hematemesis, while hematochezia can also be seen in patients who are bleeding heavily. Since 2–10% of peptic ulcers are complicated by perforations, patients who experience abrupt, intense, diffuse abdominal discomfort should be suspected of having an ulcer perforation (Di Saverio et al., 2014).

Patients with perforations may experience abrupt abdominal discomfort in the early hours following the onset, which often starts in the epigastric region and quickly spreads to the rest of the body. Both shoulders or the top of the right shoulder may experience radiating pain. There are moments when the pain is so intense that it can cause syncope or collapse. Moreover, tachycardia, a weak pulse, and low temperature are caused by gastric acid irritating the peritoneal cavity. Abdominal discomfort may gradually become more extensive. Examination of the patient may reveal board-like rigidity of the abdomen and obliteration of liver dullness because of peritoneal air. A rectal examination may indicate pelvic peritoneum pain as a result of accumulated inflammatory fluid. Symptoms may be far less acute if the peritoneum or retroperitoneal perforation limits the leak and gastric fluid flow to a small area. Compared to free intraperitoneal perforation, the upper abdominal pain in retroperitoneal perforation is more delicate, and the abdominal examination is sometimes ambiguous. There is a temporal delay in the onset of stomach pain associated with retroperitoneal perforation. It is imperative to diagnose perforations as soon as possible since postponing treatment might lead to the progression of peritonitis, which can induce hypovolemia, elevated body temperature, and cardiovascular collapse. The least common PUD complication, gastric outlet or duodenal channel ulceration, is gastric outlet obstruction (GOO). As the incidence of PUD declines, cancer is now the most common cause of GOO. Early satiety, bloating, indigestion, nausea, vomiting, epigastric discomfort, anorexia, and weight loss are among the signs and symptoms of GOO.

1.11. Tests and Diagnosis

To accurately detect *H. pylori* infection, invasive, and noninvasive diagnostic techniques have been employed since it was identified as a factor in the development of peptic ulcers. Esophagogastroduodenoscopy (EGD) (Figure 1.10) or upper endoscopy and biopsy are necessary as invasive techniques (Otuya et al., 2018). These procedures are then followed by a culture of the bacteria, a rapid urease test (RUT), molecular testing (PCR), or histological evaluation (fluorescence *in situ* hybridization-FISH). Additional diagnostic procedures include non-invasive techniques like the stool antigen test (SAT), the urea breath test (UBT), and serological testing for the identification of *H. pylori* antibodies.

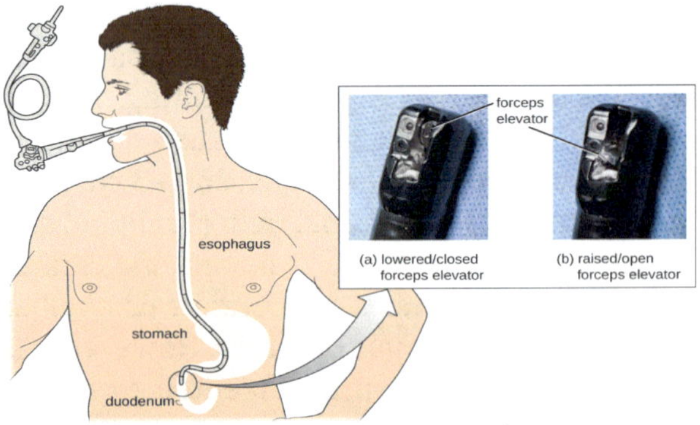

Figure 1.10. *Esophagogastroduodenoscopy.*

Source: https://upload.wikimedia.org/wikipedia/commons/2/24/OSC_Microbio_13_04_DuoScope.jpg, Creative Commons License.

Noninvasive diagnostics can occasionally be used as a substitute for EGD, which helps to reduce the effort and cost. The degree to which a patient experiences symptoms determines the diagnosis of peptic ulcer disease. Testing for *H. pylori* antibiotic susceptibility in stomach biopsy tissues is crucial for determining the treatment. It is important to determine whether the patient needs an upper endoscopy for evaluation, weigh the benefits of this approach versus less invasive techniques, and determine whether the risks outweigh any potential benefits for the patient. For the diagnosis of *H. pylori* in adults, there is no gold standard technique. The selection of the diagnostic test is extremely individualized and is contingent upon the clinical context, pre-test chance of infection, usage of recent or current drugs, as well as the diagnostic test's local availability and cost. It is important to note that antibiotics, also known as proton pump inhibitors (PPIs), lower bacterial density, impact test sensitivity, and lower test accuracy for active infection.

Many investigations have been carried out to evaluate the efficacy of distinct PPIs in managing duodenal ulcers, gastric ulcers, and gastric ulcers associated with NSAIDs. There is substantial evidence that omeprazole (20 mg) and lansoprazole (20 mg) are equally beneficial for curing duodenal ulcer symptoms and promoting healing. There was no discernible difference in the induction of duodenal ulcer healing between pantoprazole (40 mg) and rabeprazole (20 mg) when compared with omeprazole (20 mg). Research has also demonstrated that one week of omeprazole and antibiotic therapy is just as successful in curing duodenal ulcers as the suggested regimen of one week of omeprazole and antibiotic therapy followed by three weeks of PPI therapy. Patients who are regularly taking NSAIDs for arthritic disorders did not exhibit a statistically significant difference in remission rates between pantoprazole (40 mg) and omeprazole (20 mg).

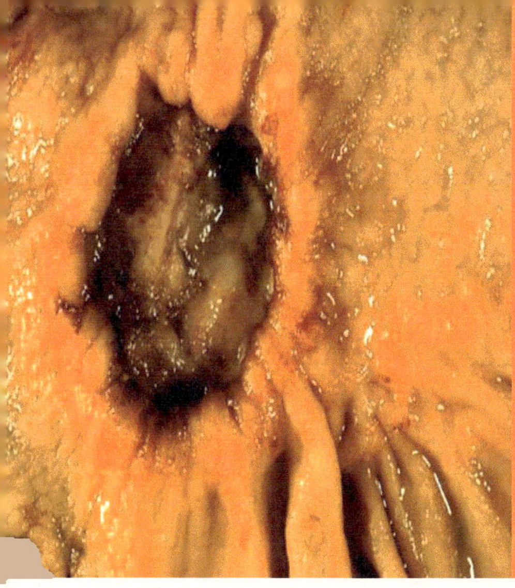

Chapter 2

GI DISEASES AND NUTRITION

Contents

2.1. Introduction

Some decades ago, medical teams were said to have a difficult time identifying hospital malnutrition, despite its high prevalence. Protein calorie malnutrition (PCM) is still a common condition among hospitalized patients, and many doctors still do not fully understand it. 48% of hospitalized patients in Brazil were found to be malnourished (Pirlich and Lochs, 2001). The majority of doctors did not evaluate their patients' nutritional condition or include nutritional therapy as a primary part of their treatment. When PCM affects the physiologic capabilities, hinders one's response to medical therapy, or lengthens the time it takes for an individual to recover, it becomes clinically significant. The loss of all body protein and muscle function is what causes the physiologic degradation associated with PCM. Significant impairments occur in physiologic body functions when a patient loses more than 20% of their normal body weight. Research assessing the connection between body protein loss and weight loss has demonstrated a correlation. Malnutrition has a negative effect on organ function. There are two broad kinds of protein malnutrition: kwashiorkor (Figure 2.1) and marasmus.

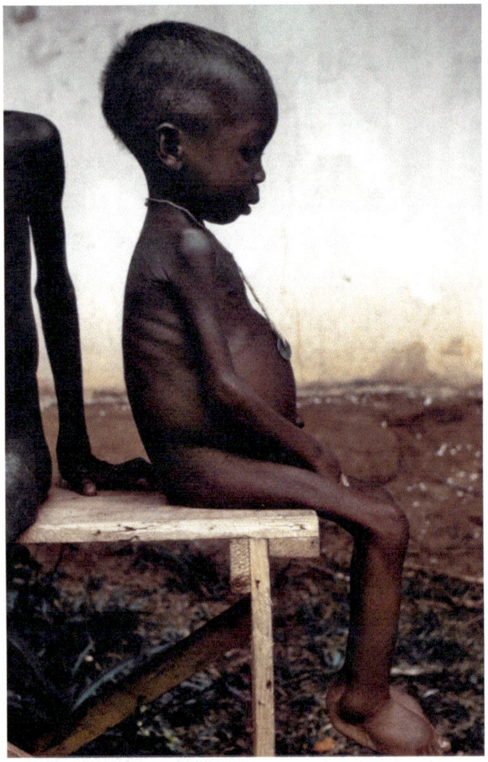

Figure 2.1. *Kwashiorkor.*

Source: https://upload.wikimedia.org/wikipedia/commons/4/47/Starved_girl.jpg, Creative Commons License.

Individuals diagnosed with marasmus exhibit a prominent reduction in total body fat and body protein, accompanied by a minor increase in extracellular water. In a clinical setting, this manifests as body wasting. The cheekbones and skull may protrude, and the eyes may be sunken. A low normal range is frequently found in the plasma albumin. Despite severe physiological dysfunction, these patients do not exhibit an increase in resting energy expenditure. Individuals suffering from kwashiorkor exhibit comparable deficiencies in body fat and protein, but they also exhibit a prominent rise in extracellular fluid and a decrease in plasma albumin levels. This extracellular fluid increase may appear to be masking underlying weight loss to an untrained eye. In addition to having an elevated metabolic rate, patients with kwashiorkor would also have reduced physiological function. Over time, muscle strength declines due to malnutrition. Peak expiratory flow forced expiratory volume, and vital capacity all decrease with respiratory function. It has been reported that malnutrition and poor respiratory gas exchange are associated in individuals with chronic obstructive pulmonary disease. In addition, malnutrition can weaken the immune system, decrease cardiac output, and impede wound healing.

2.2. Nutrition and Its Status

Nutritional repletion therapy frequently stops these deteriorating processes and greatly enhances patient outcomes. In addition to treating these diseases, the challenge is identifying those who are at risk so that the right interventions can be implemented. The field of nutrition assessment research is still evolving. Early studies on determining if malnutrition is present led to the development of techniques and markers for quickly surveying huge populations. After that, a large number of these tools and indicators were introduced to the hospital environment and applied to specific patients. Serum albumin is one of the commonly used conventional indicators of protein-calorie malnutrition, however, its high variance and low sensitivity make it useless for use in treating individual patients (Briassoulis, 2014). A medical, nutritional, and body weight history are frequently included in a standard nutrition assessment. Current body weight and height measurements are kept on file. The total final examination may include serum protein levels, body anthropometric measurements, immune competence efficacy, and functional measurements of muscular strength. When taken separately, these metrics frequently do not provide enough information to reliably assess a patient's nutrition risk. Instead of taking a precise weight, the majority of doctors and nurses rely on patients' recollections of their own weight, which is an extremely unreliable method. Research has repeatedly shown that no single tool or method of assessment is sufficient to determine the nutritional status of a patient. To improve our sensitivity and specificity in assessing nutritional status, combinations of several metrics have been created into scoring systems. Global approaches to hospitalized patient nutrition assessment can often give a significantly more accurate picture of the patient's nutrition risk.

2.3. Anthropometrics

The scientific study of human body measurements is called anthropometrics (Figure 2.2) (Steckel, 2024). Body compartment measurements can be used to assess the body energy stores. Two bedside tools, a Lange^R caliper and tape measure, are employed in anthropometrics as a bedside technique for assessing body fat and protein reserves. Anthropometric measurements can be compared to reference values and then monitored over time in the same subject. Anthropometrics' dependence on age, sex, and race-matched reference data is a disadvantage. Bedridden patients may have a drop in muscle mass without a matching fall in body protein stores since muscle mass is largely reliant on exercise. Anthropometric techniques frequently yield inaccurate assessments of body protein and fat reserves in several patients. Patients in critical condition, as well as those with liver, kidney, or both, frequently exhibit severe edema and an increase in bodily fluids.

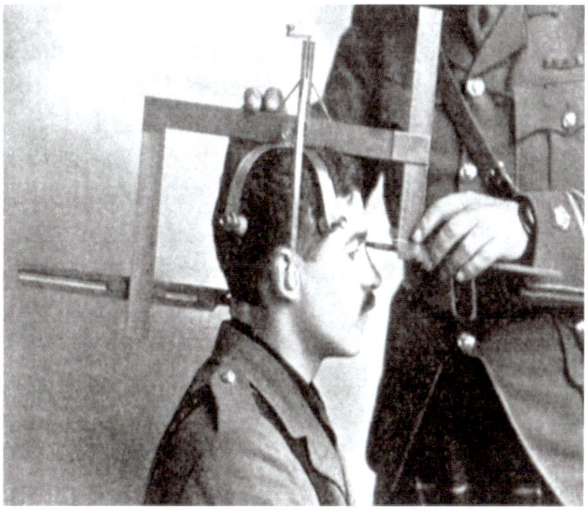

Figure 2.2. *Anthropometrics.*

Source: https://upload.wikimedia.org/wikipedia/commons/3/34/Head-Measurer_of_Tremearne_%28side_view%29.jpg, Creative Commons License.

There is a substantial variation in anthropometric measurements made by different clinicians on the same patient, with reports ranging from 5 to 23%. It has been established that the triceps skinfold, measured using a Lange^R caliper, is an indirect indicator of body fat storage. It has also been established that midarm muscle circumference (MAMC), which is measured with a tape at the midpoint of the upper arm, serves as an indirect indicator of body protein storage. Between 900 mm^2 and 1200 mm^2 is the minimal MAMC. A BMI < 20 kg/m^2 and a MAMC below the 15th percentile are commonly used to define malnutrition (Joosten et al.,1999). Nutritional markers include plasma proteins, such as albumin, ferritin, prealbumin, transferrin, and retinol-binding protein. The intravascular compartment retains one-third of albumin, while the extravascular compartment holds the remaining two-thirds. Albumin synthesis and degradation or losses in the liver are both represented by serum albumin levels. The overall body water status, liver function, and renal losses of a patient influence the blood concentrations of albumin and other plasma proteins. Serum proteins are supposedly accurate nutritional markers; however, they are really better understood as indicators of a patient's general health rather than as actual nutritional markers. The degree of hypoalbuminemia (Figure 2.3) and the 30-day death rate (mortality) among hospitalized patients were found to be linearly correlated (Reinhardt et al., 1980). Old patients undergoing heart surgery who had low serum albumin levels also had an increase in inpatient (hospital) mortality. Research has demonstrated that clinical judgment based on a patient's medical history and physical examination is a more sensitive indication of a nutritional state than serum albumin. The degree and importance of malnutrition can be determined by taking direct measures of body functioning. For instance, malnutrition can quickly impair skeletal muscle function independent of other serious medical conditions including sepsis, trauma, or renal failure. Standardized force-frequency curves have been obtained. A handgrip dynamometer, a bedside device, can be used to assess muscle mass from handgrip strength in a patient who can obey directions. It has been demonstrated that hospitalized patients with weak grip strength have longer hospital stays, are less able to return home, and have higher mortality rates. Individuals suffering from Crohn's disease and ulcerative colitis may have significant changes in their nutritional condition. Reduced food intake, digestion, and absorption; changed nutrient metabolism and drug-nutrient interactions can all contribute to this. Dietary factors have also been linked to the development of IBD. Some dietary therapies might emerge in the future if it is discovered that nutrients are possible immunomodulators in these diseases. Crohn's disease and ulcerative colitis are the two most prevalent diagnoses associated with intestinal inflammation that make up the category of inflammatory bowel disease. Malnutrition is linked to these diseases, which include shortages in vitamins, minerals, and protein-calorie intake. As efforts to identify the etiologies of these diseases have been undertaken, several eating habits have been linked. The goals of nutritional assistance for patients with inflammatory bowel disease have been to address growth failure, nutritional inadequacies, and act as a main therapy.

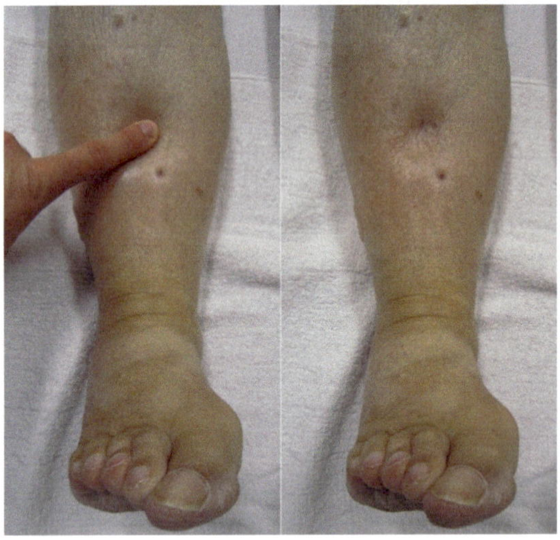

Figure 2.3. *Hypoalbuminemia.*

Source: https://upload.wikimedia.org/wikipedia/commons/8/84/Combinpedal.jpg, Creative Commons License.

2.4. Inflammatory Bowel Disease

Over the years, inflammatory bowel disease and nutrition have been reviewed extensively.

These differ in how they manage Crohn's disease nutritionally based on whether the reports were written in Europe or the United States. Like many other gastrointestinal disorders, inflammatory bowel disease (IBD) can have an impact on a person's nutritional health. Dietary habits may have a part in the pathophysiology of certain intestinal diseases. The nutrition and dietary modification may change how the disease progresses.

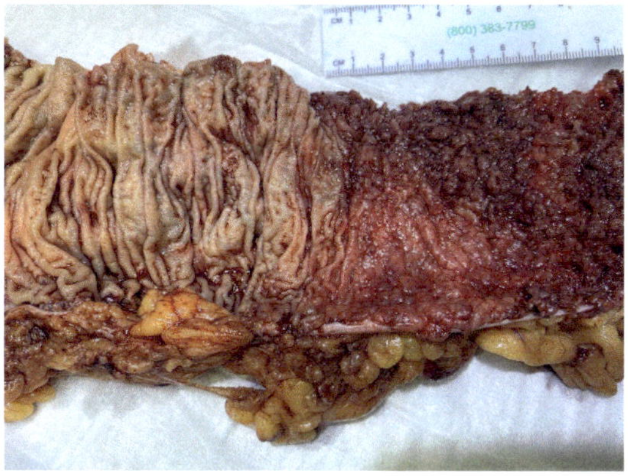

Figure 2.4. *Pancolitis.*

Source: https://upload.wikimedia.org/wikipedia/commons/1/1b/Severe_ulcerative_colitis.jpg, Creative Commons License.

These diagnoses include the majority of inflammatory disorders of the small intestine and colon, even though they only make up a minor number of the disease states grouped together under the umbrella of IBD. Any area of the gastrointestinal system, from the mouth to the anus, can be impacted by Crohn's disease. This is a transmural disease that affects 35–45% of cases in the terminal ileum and colon, only 25–35% in the terminal ileum, only 15–25% in the colon, and 5–10% in the proximal small bowel (Goulart et al., 2016). The common form of Crohn's disease is skip lesions with scattered normal mucosa. Before the last decades, the pillars of treatment were corticosteroids and surgical resection; however, more modern treatments utilizing immunomodulating medications (drugs) have prioritized both reducing steroid therapy problems and conserving the intestine loss during resection. Globally, the prevalence of Crohn's disease is increasing. Ulcerative colitis affects primarily the colon and can occasionally be accompanied by backwash ileitis, which affects the terminal ileum. It is distinguished by persistent inflammatory alterations in the colon, extending from the rectum to the proximal end. Usually, it just affects the intestinal mucosal and submucosal layers. About 20% of cases have pancolitis (Figure 2.4).

2.5. Important Characteristics of Crohn's Disease

There are distinctions in the anatomical and pathophysiology characteristics of Crohn's disease (CD) and ulcerative colitis (UC) that affect the consequences (symptoms) for nutritional status in people with IBD. The mechanisms behind malnutrition can be broadly classified into some groups in almost all disease conditions. These include reduced food intake, poor digestion, malabsorption, changes in the way nutrients are metabolized, higher nutrient needs, higher nutrient losses, and interactions between drugs and nutrients. Reduced food consumption is a common occurrence in IBD, particularly in Crohn's disease. This often happens as a result of anorexia, the correlation between food consumption and symptoms such as nausea, vomiting, diarrhea, or discomfort, as well as the application of different restrictive diets by different people for different purposes. Recent studies have looked into the potential connection between proinflammatory cytokines and IBD-related anorexia. Some researchers reported increased 5-hydroxytryptamine (5-HT) release from the hypothalamus paraventricular nucleus in a rat model of colitis. When p-chlorophenyl alanine was injected into the hypothalamus to deplete brain 5-HT, the food intake returned to normal, although it had dropped in comparison to healthy controls. Some years ago, it was demonstrated that injecting interleukin-1 (IL-1) increased the release of 5-HT from the hypothalamus (Figure 2.5). It has been shown that leptins reduce food intake. It is also commonly known that proinflammatory cytokines, such as interleukin 6 (IL-6), tumor necrosis factor-alpha (TNF-α), and IL-1, are elevated in active Crohn's disease and that they contribute to the pathophysiology of IBD. These results point to a potential connection between IBD anorexia and pro-inflammatory cytokines.

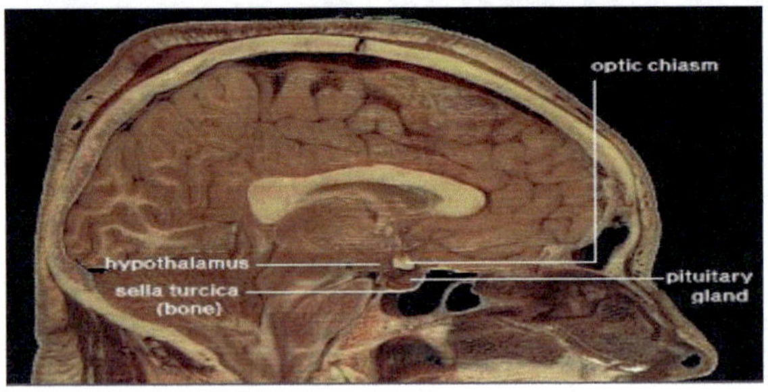

Figure 2.5. *Hypothalamus.*

Source: https://upload.wikimedia.org/wikipedia/commons/9/9f/LocationOfHypothalamus.jpg, Creative Commons License.

Sensations like nausea, discomfort, diarrhea, and incontinence that the patient associates with eating may limit their intake of food. Moreover, it is common for the clinician to discover that patients have restricted their food intake due to diets prescribed by various sources, including the medical community, family, and the Internet in recent times. It happens frequently that patients discover whole food groups have been cut out of their diet after receiving several recommendations to reduce a range of foods. It has been demonstrated that the dietary views of patients with IBD can drastically change their eating habits, especially when it comes to consuming less calcium and folic acid. Food consumed may be lacking in some nutrients as a result of these unique dietary guidelines. Nutrient maldigestion may result from the damaged mucosa in small intestine Crohn's disease cases (Montoro-Huguet et al., 2021). This can happen in proximal disease when mucosal damage destroys mucosal disaccharidases, allowing undigested carbohydrates to create osmotic loads and generating diarrhea and flatulence due to colonic flora metabolism.

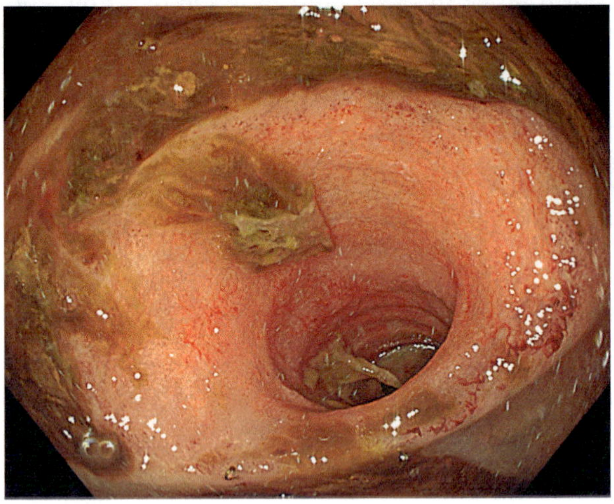

Figure 2.6. *Ileal disease.*

Source: https://upload.wikimedia.org/wikipedia/commons/1/12/Ileitis_AO_AL.jpg, Creative Commons License.

Ileal disease (Figure 2.6) may lead to a reduction in the amount of bile acid absorbed, which would lower the bile acid pool. Because triglycerides and pancreatic enzymes are not sufficiently mixed, lipids cannot be solubilized and are thus poorly digested in the lumen of the proximal small bowel. Decreased bile output as well as decreased fat and fat-soluble vitamin digestion and absorption might be consequences of primary sclerosing cholangitis, a biliary complication of IBD, particularly ulcerative colitis. Due to bacterial deconjugation of bile salts, small intestine bacterial overgrowth may also result in fat maldigestion. The small intestine's expanded and changed flora cause gradual mucosal injury and disaccharidases to be depleted. Inflammation of the intestinal mucosa and intestinal resection, which reduces the mucosal surface area accessible for absorption, are the main causes of malabsorption, particularly in Crohn's disease. The absorption of bile acids (along with vitamin B_{12}) is impacted by distal ileal resection. Because of the bacterial preferred consumption of vitamin B_{12} and the resulting depletion of the B_{12} supply accessible to the distal ileum, bacterial overgrowth also results in malabsorption of vitamin B_{12}. The problem of malabsorption is less common in ulcerative colitis.

2.6. Immunological Responses

The concept of altered cytokine-mediated nutrition metabolism has emerged in recent Crohn's disease research. TNF, IL-1, and IL-6 are examples of inflammatory cytokines that are produced in response to diverse stimuli by activated monocytes/macrophages (Figure 2.7) and lymphocytes, which change the metabolism of protein, carbohydrate, and lipid. These proinflammatory cytokines are overproduced in the intestinal mucosa and blood in patients with Crohn's disease. Some researchers discovered a correlation between inflammatory cytokine levels and univariate examination of multiple anthropometric and biochemical indicators of dietary status in Crohn's disease patients. In particular, TNF levels were negatively connected with mean arm circumference (MAC), triceps skinfold thickness (TSF), transthyretin, and albumin; on the other hand, IL-1 was negatively correlated with body weight (BW), body mass index (BMI), MAC, and albumin. There was a negative correlation found between inflammatory proteins such as fibrinogen, orosomucoid, C-reactive protein, erythrocyte sedimentation rate, and transthyretin and nutritional factors including albumin and transthyretin. Positive correlations were found between albumin, transthyretin, retinol-binding protein, and vitamin A levels and insulin-like growth factor (IGF-1). Fever and sepsis in IBD patients may lead to an increased calorie need. Malnutrition has been linked to elevated basal metabolic rate in active IBD, while this is most likely not the case in quiescent disease. As those who are sick tend to be less active, the greater basal energy requirements in those with active disease are probably countered by decreased requirements for exercise. Compared to controls, patients with active Crohn's disease had higher resting energy expenditures, improved lipid oxidation, and lower diet-induced thermogenesis. Lipid peroxidation impact was closely linked to the activity of the disease. However, patients with inactive Crohn's disease were also found to have elevated lipid oxidation. In IBD, accelerated mucosal cell turnover may also result in higher dietary needs.

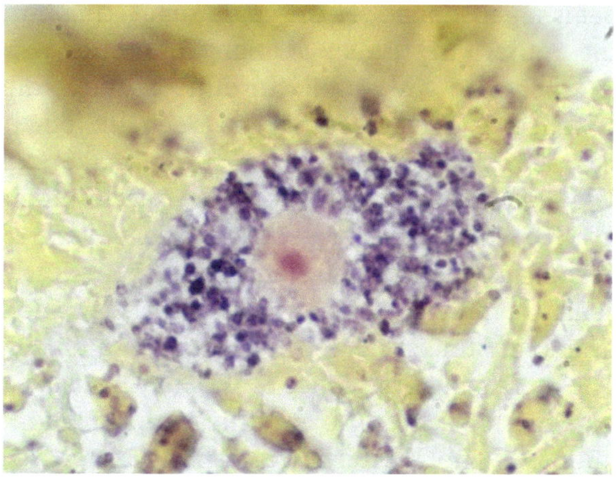

Figure 2.7. *Macrophages.*

Source: https://upload.wikimedia.org/wikipedia/commons/7/77/Gram_stain_of_a_macrophage_with_ingested_S_epidermidis_bacteria.jpg reative Commons License.

Both Crohn's disease and ulcerative colitis cause increased nutritional losses because of inflammation and protein and fluid transudation from the infected mucosa. The mucosal bleeding results in iron loss. Zinc, fluid, and electrolyte loss is brought on by fistulae, which are most frequently seen in Crohn's disease. Fats are mainly associated with Crohn's disease. Another potential cause of malnutrition in IBD patients is drug-nutrient interactions. Sulfasalazine inhibits the breakdown of folic acid into its active form, tetrahydrofolate, by decreasing the absorption of folic acid and dihydrofolate reductase (Gisondi et al., 2007). Corticosteroids change protein metabolism, impair calcium absorption, induce magnesuria, and promote muscular atrophy. The amount of vitamin K that is produced by colonic bacterial metabolism can be reduced by antibiotics. Bile acids are bound by cholestyramine and are hence inaccessible for proper fat and fat-soluble vitamin digestion. The cause of Crohn's disease and ulcerative colitis has never been fully understood, and investigations into the pathophysiology of the conditions have given rise to many theories, some of which are dietary in nature. There have been suggestions over the years suggesting that the underlying cause of many ailments was an allergy to cow's milk. In other studies, the absence of breastfeeding has been linked. It has been proposed that high sugar intake and low dietary fiber are linked to the development of IBD. It has been suggested that exposure to certain environmental elements in genetically sensitive individuals may trigger an upregulation of the immune system, which could lead to IBD. The increasing prevalence of IBD may be caused by food and lifestyle modifications brought about by the Western world. It is suggested that the intestinal lumen exposure to particular nutrients could function as an antigenic agent or as a modulator of the mucosal cell regulatory processes, which could ultimately result in inflammatory bowel disease (IBD).

2.7. Fatty Acid Biochemistry

It has long been known that colonocytes prefer short-chain fatty acids as fuel. The prevalent short-chain fatty acid in the intestinal lumen is butyrate, a 4C saturated fatty acid that is produced mostly by bacteria from unabsorbed carbohydrates, mainly dietary fiber. Some researchers discovered that in tissue cultures taken from colonic biopsies of Crohn's colitis patients, butyrate has an anti-inflammatory impact by reducing the synthesis of TNF, cytokine messenger RNA expression, and nuclear factor B. Nuclear factor B, which controls the transcription of cytokine genes, including TNF, was suggested as the last mediator. This initiates a question of whether a lower dietary fiber intake plays a factor in the development of IBD, especially in cases with colon disease. The hypothesized etiologic agent, dietary fat, has been partially linked to the decreased frequency of inflammatory diseases among Greenland Eskimos. This demographic consumes a lot of fish, which increases their intake of omega-3 fatty acids, which have anti-inflammatory properties. Some studies suggested a link between high consumption of monounsaturated fats, vitamin B_6, and omega-6 fatty acids, with a higher risk of ulcerative colitis. Malnutrition is frequently present in patients with Crohn's disease and ulcerative colitis. Early observations of Crohn's disease described weight loss in cases of regional ileitis. Up to 80% of people with Crohn's disease and as many as 50–60% of people with ulcerative colitis still exhibit protein-calorie deficiency (Javelli, 2015). Approximately 25–80% of individuals with Crohn's disease and 25–50% of patients with ulcerative colitis have hypoalbuminemia; however, it has been determined that this is mostly due to disease activity rather than a nutritional shortage.

2.8. Anemia

A significant portion of people with IBD have anemia. Usually, a shortage of iron, vitamin B_{12}, or folate causes this. More than 80% of individuals with ulcerative colitis have iron deficiency anemia, which is mostly caused by blood loss. It is observed in approximately 40% of anemic Crohn's disease patients, particularly in cases when the disease affects the colon. On the other hand, vitamin B_{12} deficiency is rare in ulcerative colitis patients; instead, it is common in patients with distal ileal Crohn's disease or a history of ileal resection. Folate deficiency is seen in one-third to half of people with IBD, with Crohn's disease having a somewhat greater frequency. 40 to 90% of patients with IBD had blood levels of biotin, folate, thiamine, vitamin A, E, C, and beta-carotene that were below the fifteenth percentile of normal (reference) controls. Clinical suspicion is crucial for keeping an eye on patients who may be at risk of developing deficient states because these were found in patients who did not show any clinical symptoms or who did not appear to be decreasing their intakes.

Deficits in fat-soluble vitamins are more common in patients with reduced bile salt pools, and cholestasis, which can cause sclerosing cholangitis and bacterial overgrowth syndrome. Because vitamin A is linked to immunological function, vitamin A deficiency has been a source of concern. There has been evidence of a higher prevalence of vitamin A deficiency in pediatric patients with both Crohn's disease and ulcerative colitis, which has been linked to the severity of the disease. Patients with IBD should be especially concerned about selenium deficiency since, along with vitamins E, A, and C, it functions as an antioxidant. The process of IBD most likely involves oxidative stress (Piechota-Polanczyk and Fichna, 2014). Serum selenium and glutathione peroxidase levels in red blood cells were shown to be lower in Crohn's disease patients. These findings led researchers to hypothesize that a selenium shortage may contribute to immunological and inflammatory activation in the condition. In Crohn's disease, magnesium shortage is very common, especially after distal small bowel resection and colectomy.

2.9. Nutritional Deficiency

Zinc deficiency is common in people with Crohn's disease and related fistulae. People who have IBD are frequently found to have metabolic bone disease. Malnutrition is undoubtedly a factor in this situation. Over 10% of people with inflammatory bowel disease have hypocalcemia (Jasielska and Grzybowska-Chlebowczyk, 2021). This is frequently linked to reduced vitamin D levels, particularly in individuals receiving corticosteroid drugs. More than half of patients with low vitamin D levels have been observed to have osteopenia. Nevertheless, recent research studies found that while parathyroid hormone and alkaline phosphatase were significantly greater, low bone mineral density (BMD) was not common in individuals with low 25-OH vitamin D levels. Reduced exposure to sunlight, poor nutritional condition (low serum iron and red blood cell folate levels), and smoking were linked to decreased 25-OH vitamin D levels in Crohn's disease patients. Winter vitamin D levels were four times lower than spring and summer levels. Crohn's disease patients experienced the clinical effects of bone disease, particularly vertebral fractures. Documenting risk factors for metabolic bone disease in IBD has been the focus of other studies. Age, body mass index, and blood magnesium levels were found to be linked with bone mineral density (BMD); however, lifetime steroid use was not a good predictor. Some researchers found that patients with Crohn's disease who, as a result of steroid sparing treatment approaches, including diet, had a low lifetime corticosteroid use, had BMD levels comparable to normal controls, and that patients who received steroids had a significantly lower BMD. Clinicians need to be aware that patients with IBD may develop osteoporosis. They also need to evaluate BMD, treat patients with calcium and vitamin D replacement when necessary, and take into account bisphosphonates in those individuals.

The patients are already at risk for nutritional loss from the start of IBD. The patients with Crohn's disease were taller than randomly selected controls from a patient database, but their body mineral content was lower. Compared to controls, those with ulcerative colitis had a higher body mass index. Compared to the control groups, patients with Crohn's disease and ulcerative colitis had higher fat free mass and lower fat free mass, respectively. Expert nutritionists conducted food intake interviews and examined data to determine the daily nutritional consumption. Based on data, it was discovered that compared to the control group, people with Crohn's disease consumed less polyunsaturated fatty acids but more mono and disaccharides. In comparison to controls, those with ulcerative colitis consumed less protein overall and less phosphorus, calcium, riboflavin, and vitamin C. Less alcohol was consumed by both patient groups than by either control group. Biochemical markers revealed that patients with ulcerative colitis had significantly lower amounts of albumin, magnesium, zinc, and beta-carotene and that those with Crohn's disease had significantly lower levels of these nutrients. Based on the CDAI (Crohn's disease activity index) and Witt's and Truelove criteria, a substantial portion of these patients were determined to be in clinical remission, respectively (Gisbert et al., 2008). The assistance of a dietitian can help identify nutrient deficiencies, indicating which dietary practices may contribute and correcting them, encouraging patients to follow recommendations, and monitoring the patient, provided the doctor has the specialized training in nutrition and the time to adequately address these issues. To establish effective approaches to correction with the diet itself, as well as the use of calorie supplements and specialized drugs, inadequate protein and calorie intakes require an understanding of the constraints in individual patients.

2.10. Vitamins

For people with specific deficiencies of vitamins A, D, E, and K, the availability of a chewable multivitamin comprising the water-soluble forms of the fat-soluble vitamins is often beneficial. However, very high doses of ergocalciferol are typically required to achieve the 25-OH vitamin D levels considered necessary to treat osteoporosis. It is important to remember that when using such high dosages, blood levels of the vitamin must be monitored to ensure that hypervitaminosis does not develop. It is now known that oral dosing with very high doses of cyanocobalamin will effectively replace the vitamin in many patients with low levels of B_{12} due to passive absorption of up to 10% of the dose. It is crucial to keep an eye on blood levels to ensure that a patient receiving oral replacement therapy is receiving enough of it. In patients with Crohn's disease, higher homocysteine levels have been linked to lower folate levels. This implies that to reduce coronary artery disease and deep vein thrombosis, vitamin replacement should be prioritized. Folate supplementation may prevent dysplasia from developing in IBD patient intestinal mucosa. Zinc supplements are a readily available means of replacing minerals, particularly zinc. The difficulty in replacing magnesium is to offer a magnesium salt that does not result in catharsis. Organic magnesium salts, such as magnesium gluconate, which comes in tablet or elixir form, are an effective way to replace magnesium. Because these organic salts dissociate gradually in solution, the osmotic burden is reduced and therapeutic efficacy is enhanced. Crohn's disease may persist due to subclinical deficiencies. Lipid peroxidation may be stimulated by defects in tissue repair systems that lead to a weakened defense against damage from oxygen free radicals. The concept that IBD may put stress on antioxidant vitamin levels is important. This clearly implies that physicians need to pay close attention to patient diets and nutritional conditions and that primary nutritional therapy might play a part in maintaining remission. The treatment objective for inflammatory bowel disease (IBD) is to down-regulate the immune response to heal bowel lesions and hence improve symptoms and quality of life, with minimal side effects. Pharmacologic treatments for IBD, both those used in the past and those being used now, are linked to adverse effects. This suggests that food modification could be a safe substitute or perhaps an additional strategy to lessen reliance on different immunomodulatory drugs. This should be taken into account, particularly for individuals who may require steroids in the long run, those who are resistant to, intolerant of, or dependent on steroids and other drugs, those who are particularly at risk for osteoporosis, and those who ask for other forms of treatment. However, an assessment should be conducted before initiating a food regimen to ascertain whether the patient is likely to comply due to treatment acceptability issues or inconvenience.

2.11. Cancer

Nutritional status can be greatly impacted by gastrointestinal diseases. Research shows that malnutrition has a detrimental effect on cancer patients' quality of life (QOL), survival rate, and reaction to treatment. Patients with gastrointestinal cancer should receive nutritional assistance, which may vary depending on their anticancer therapy strategy. In some conditions, parenteral nutrition, enteral nutrition, and immunonutrition interventions are appropriate. Changing one's diet may also be crucial for preventing cancer. Approximately 20% of all malignancies and cancer-related deaths in the US occur from gastrointestinal cancers each year (Arnold et al., 2020). In the US, colorectal cancer is the third most prevalent cause of cancer-related deaths and the fourth most common type of cancer overall. The impact of gastrointestinal diseases on body composition, weight, and quality of life can be long-lasting. It is critical to provide adequate nutrition before, during, and after therapy. It is crucial to take into account the ways in which dietary variables may affect the risk of GI cancer. The development of cancer typically takes decades and can be activated by the combined effects of several different variables. This not only complicates the pertinent pathways but also makes it challenging to identify specific dietary causes of cancer. Moreover, it is rarely possible to identify a specific cancer dietary etiology. The processes of food carcinogenesis have been explained by both *in vitro* and *in vivo* research. Understanding the biochemical and molecular relationships between nutrition and cancer depends heavily on *in vitro* research.

Oncogene mutations (Figure 2.8) are essential for the development of cancer, and *in-vitro* research has demonstrated the potential impact that dietary components may have in the production of these mutations. Food-based compounds may provide protection against these changes. Theories about the biological impact of food and food-based chemicals on GI carcinogenesis are aided by the use of animal models. The mechanisms of carcinogenesis and cancer prevention may be tested in animal models. Experiments requiring precisely defined nutritional treatments under closely monitored conditions can be designed due to animal systems. However, because of species differences, these results cannot be directly applied to humans. The main source of knowledge about how foods and dietary ingredients affect cancer risk is epidemiologic research. Nevertheless, not all confounding factors can be controlled for in these investigations. In addition to having an impact on carcinogenesis, exposure to exogenous and endogenous carcinogens such as radiation, physical agents, microbes, and viruses can also make it more difficult to analyze data collected from epidemiological studies. While case-control and human dietary intervention studies offer more precise data, they are costly and challenging to do. It takes years for specific sets of nutritional theories to be tested in interventional diet experiments (trials). It is unclear if a specific nutrient efficacy is tumor-specific or dependent on a critical exposure period. The reliability of diet-type observations is higher than that of food or nutrient-specific observations. In human dietary trials, specific nutrients like beta-carotene, vitamin E, and vitamin A that were previously reported to be protective through epidemiologic research are ineffective or even unsafe when supplemented. This could be the result of several factors such as the nutrients being separated from the entire food source, or it could be caused by population-specific traits. Fruits and vegetables contain a range of healthy chemicals, many of which probably combine to produce positive effects. Whole foods may contain significant but hidden ingredients that are left out of specific supplements. There is not much proof that dietary supplements can replace the advantages of a carefully planned, nutrient-enriched diet.

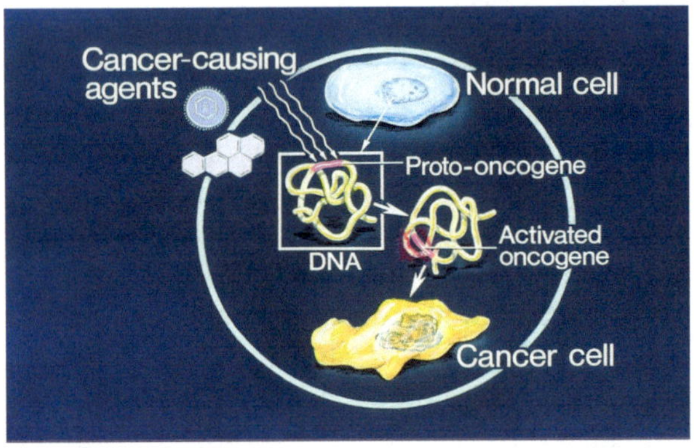

Figure 2.8. *Oncogene mutations.*

Source: https://upload.wikimedia.org/wikipedia/commons/d/de/Oncogenes_illustration.jpg, Creative Commons License.

Dietary variables that increase the risk of cancer include a sedentary lifestyle, excessive energy intake, and certain foods (Kerr et al., 2017). The risk and death of cancer are positively linked with energy intake. It is interesting to note that real energy expenditure and energy intake have a considerable impact on cancer risk, but elevated BMI, an indicator of obesity and thus a substitution for excessive energy consumption, does not appear to influence risk. Direct DNA damage (nitrites), cytochrome activation or inhibition (alcohol), carcinogen activation (pickles/salted foods), direct cytotoxicity (mycotoxins), oxidative damage (saturated fats), changes in physiology (rice, dietary fiber), and hormonal effects (phytoestrogens) are some of the mechanisms of dietary carcinogenesis. Many dietary components have been proposed as precautionary against esophageal cancer, including zinc, vitamin C, green tea, and fruits and vegetables. It is hypothesized that fruits and vegetables influence the natural antioxidant mechanisms and reduce the synthesis of nitrosamines. Dietary fiber and phytochemical intake are linked to suboptimal fruit and vegetable consumption. Fiber is crucial for the sequestration and evacuation of procarcinogens from the colon and rectum, whereas phytochemicals may help prevent stomach cancer. Epigallocatechin gallate or EGCG, the main ingredient in green tea, appears to have multiple modes of action, such as intracellular antioxidant, procarcinogen production inhibition, angiogenesis, and cancer cell proliferation reduction, and so on. Drinking green tea may provide protection from the onset of some GI diseases, including esophageal cancer (Borrelli et al., 2004). Some dietary factors that have been connected to a higher risk of esophageal cancer are fat, alcohol, red meat, and simple carbohydrates. Procarcinogens and carcinogens can be found in foods that have been smoked, broiled, charred, or that are high in nitrites. One of the main ways that people are exposed to polycyclic aromatic hydrocarbons (PAHs), a family of toxicants that can be found in cigarette smoke and contaminated food, is through diet. In lab animals, PAHs are extremely carcinogenic, which may have consequences for human breast, lung, and colon cancers. Red meat consumption and simple carbohydrate intake have been connected to the synthesis of nitrosamines, a potentially carcinogenic substance. Eating more red meat and fat in the diet is linked to consuming more heterocyclic amines, another potential procarcinogen.

The risk of gastric or stomach cancer (Figure 2.9) and *H. pylori* infections are positively correlated. A large number of the food ingredients were linked to gastric chemoprotection work by regulating the *H.pylori* infection. For instance, vitamin C antioxidant properties and wine acidity seem to prevent *H. pylori* from growing. Simple carbohydrates, red meat, alcohol, and so on all seem to raise the risk of stomach cancer. By functioning as co-carcinogens in the stomach, pickles, and other salty foods raise the risk of cancer by causing oxidative stress, which in turn triggers lipid peroxidation and cellular proliferation. Consumption of fruits, vegetables, and green tea is linked to a lower risk. Dietary components linked to pancreatic cancer can also have an impact on diabetes mellitus and pancreatitis. For instance, consuming too much alcohol raises the risk of pancreatitis, which in turn raises the risk of pancreatic cancer. Consuming too many simple carbohydrates might worsen hyperglycemia in those who are vulnerable, and diabetes increases the risk of developing pancreatic cancer. Food components seem to have very little effect on liver carcinogenesis, except for alcohol-related cirrhosis. Aflatoxin exposure, cirrhosis, and HBV seem to have an impact on carcinogenesis. There is evidence that certain micronutrients, including calcium, vitamin D, folate, and selenium, have colorectal chemopreventive effects. Colon epithelial hyperproliferation brought on by bile and fatty acids is reduced by calcium, while vitamin D appears to moderate the effects of calcium. Methyl tetrahydrofolate reductase activity and the donation of methyl groups are both dependent on folate. It seems that supplementing with folate has a preventive effect on people who do not have cancer; on the other hand, it may raise the risk of cancer in those who have neoplastic tissue. Selenium stimulates coloncyte apoptosis and increases the peroxidation-inhibiting enzyme glutathione peroxidase, which may protect against colon carcinogenesis. High dietary fat consumption has been linked to an increased risk of colon cancer. The process involves the elevated secretion of primary bile acids by diet fat, which are then transformed by colonic bacteria into more cytotoxic secondary and tertiary bile acids. While early research suggested a connection between a high dietary fat intake and cancer, several epidemiologic studies conducted more recently have found little to no evidence of this relationship.

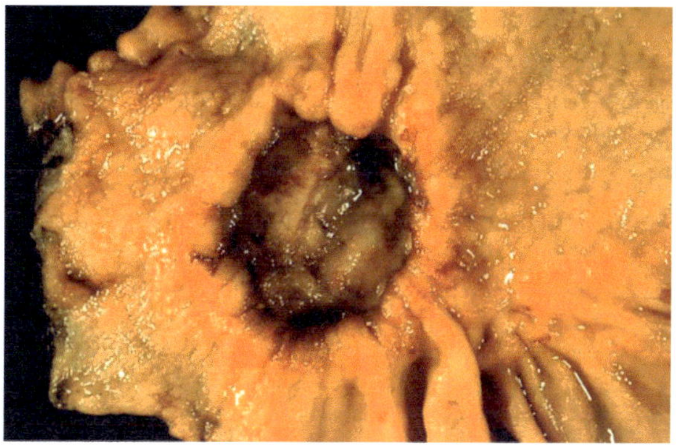

Figure 2.9. *Stomach cancer.*

Source: https://upload.wikimedia.org/wikipedia/commons/9/94/Adenocarcinoma_of_the_stomach.jpg, Creative Commons License.

Depending on the location and stage of the tumor, the prevalence of malnourishment and weight loss in patients with gastrointestinal cancers varies from 40% to 87% (Bossi et al., 2021). Pre-treatment weight loss is a poor predictive factor for patients with gastrointestinal cancers. Individuals suffering from advanced gastrointestinal cancers frequently see significant reductions in their protein and muscle composition, along with a 30%–40% fall in body fat. In four weeks, patients with solid tumors may lose up to 1.34 kg of fat-free mass. Patients with cancer who have GI diseases and lose lean body mass are more likely to encounter surgical complications. The weight loss seen in cancer patients is caused by a variety of reasons. The physiologic problems linked to the tumor, including malabsorption, obstruction, diarrhea, and vomiting, can be the reasons for weight loss; these mechanisms are particularly important in individuals with gastrointestinal malignancies. Anorexia and altered metabolism can result from host reactions to the presence of a tumor, especially when cytokines are produced. Anorexia and GI problems are also exacerbated by side effects of anti-cancer medications. For instance, individuals who get radiation therapy to the pelvis or abdomen may experience acute or chronic radiation enteritis, which can cause obstructive symptoms and/or diarrhea. Early in the course of cancer, weight alterations can be brought on by gastrointestinal and oral symptoms. Weight loss can also be caused by discomfort, anxiety, and fatigue. Anorexia, skeletal muscular atrophy, anemia, and hypoalbuminemia that are not responsive to vigorous dietary management are among the clinical characteristics of cancer cachexia. A variety of physiological and metabolic abnormalities combine to cause potentially fatal malnutrition in patients with cancer cachexia syndrome (CCS). Tumor necrosis factor (TNF), interferon (IFN), and interleukins (IL) 1 and 6, in particular, are known to trigger the development of certain symptoms linked to cachexia, including early satiety and anorexia, as well as abnormalities in the metabolism of proteins, carbohydrates, and fats. Though frequently observed in patients with cancers, CCS can exist at the start of tumor formation and potentially function as the iatrotropic stimulus. The prognostic relevance of weight loss emphasizes the need for CCS. Patients who have weight loss before treatment have a worse survival rate for any given tumor type. The best chance to avoid the effects of CCS may be to identify it early and take action to stop it from getting worse. Nutrition screening and assessment are essential for the early detection of malnutrition and CCS.

2.12. Other Aspects of Cancer

Malnutrition and weight loss are two significant factors contributing to cancer symptoms (Van Cutsem and Arends, 2005). It is particularly crucial to remember that inadequate intake is rarely the primary factor contributing to cancer-induced weight loss while dealing with cancer patients. Even when intravenously fed patients consume appropriate or even supraphysiologic amounts of calories, they typically lose weight. CCS is a metabolic condition that impacts substrate use and intermediary metabolism in addition to starvation. Therefore, unless there is a strategy in place to treat both the obstruction and the underlying cancer, it is rarely practical to undertake specialized nutrition assistance for anorexia or even GI obstruction, especially in patients with primary GI tract malignancies. No controlled studies have been conducted to support the concept that any particular dietary modifications can help treat cancer. Numerous diets, including the Gonzalez protocol, Gerson therapy, and the macrobiotic diet, make the questionable claim that they can cure cancer; however, there is no proof to support these claims. In order to prevent malnutrition in cancer patients, dietary interventions that may be helpful should focus on maintaining an adequate intake of calories and protein. A cancer patient's nutritional state can impact their quality of life, likelihood of complications, and ability to tolerate treatment. In cancer patients, enteral nutrition (EN) has been linked to improvements in the balance of nitrogen and occasionally to weight gain. PN has been linked to improvements in the balance of nitrogen in the body, and it seems to stimulate weight gain more regularly. The main cause of this weight gain, though, is body fat, and it has minimal advantages other than enhancing patient comfort and well-being. When given for 7–49 days, neither EN nor PN has a positive impact on blood proteins like albumin in cancer patients. Due to the significant importance of the underlying metabolic imbalances caused by CCS, specialized nutrition support or SNS appears to benefit cancer patients less than non-cancer patients. There has been some reluctance to utilize SNS in cancer patients due to uncertainties that supplying nutrients could promote tumor growth and metastasis. In mouse models, researchers have discovered that providing PN above energy requirements more than doubles the rate of tumor growth. Patients with colorectal cancer who are taking PN have been shown to have increased tumor cell proliferation and protein production; nevertheless, it is doubtful that this is clinically significant.

When a patient is expected to be unable to meet their nutritional needs orally for longer than 7–10 days, or when their cancer or cancer therapy has left them moderately or severely malnourished, and when future active therapy is planned to treat the underlying malignancy, then the use of SNS in cancer patients should generally be reserved. Patients receiving radiation or chemotherapy for cancer should not always be given PN. According to ASPEN standards, parenteral nutrition (PN) should only be administered to malnourished patients who are expected to have insufficient absorption of nutrients for an extended period, which is defined as more than seven to 10 days. In most situations, PN should be avoided if a patient's anticipated life expectancy is 40–60 days or less. Hydration therapy with intravenous fluids alone is advised if intravenous therapy is deemed appropriate for a patient with a life expectancy of fewer than 40 days (Miller, Raghunathan, and Gan, 2014). Many studies compared the effects of parenteral nutrition (PN) and enteral nutrition (EN) on cancer patients undergoing elective surgical resections. Perioperative PN supplementation has been shown in early studies to lower morbidity and death in cancer patients, particularly in those with gastrointestinal malignancies. The inclusion of diverse groups, inconsistent, and probably inadequate macronutrient supply, and small sample numbers have drawn criticism for these research studies. More recent perioperative parenteral nutrition (PN) studies, mainly including GI cancer patients, show no gain in survival but an increased risk of infection in these patients.

2.13. Surgery and Nutrition

After surgery, enteral feeding is typically well tolerated, and problems can usually be resolved by temporarily reducing the pace at which the enteral formula is infused. Research shows that EN is superior to PN. Early meta-analyses suggested that EN was more cost-effective than PN. Compared to the PN, studies show reduced intestinal permeability and a lower incidence of hyperglycemia. Patients with a functional gastrointestinal tract who are expected to be unable to satisfy their nutritional demands orally for a duration of seven to 10 days may benefit from perioperative EN. In oncology care, SNS intolerance is frequently a problem. Studies show that when PN is used postoperatively instead of EN, the incidence of diarrhea, distention, vomiting, and other adverse effects is reduced. Bowel rest has been advised to encourage anastomotic healing and avoid nausea and vomiting after GI surgical procedures and oral and enteral feeding has been discouraged. It has recently been established that most patients' GI function returns quickly after surgery, and intraluminal nutrients encourage intestinal hypertrophy and anastomotic recovery. Following surgery, the small intestine rapidly regains its capacity to absorb nutrition, even in the absence of peristalsis. In postoperative patients who are malnourished, early enteral feeding is linked to better immune system performance, wound healing, and gut function maintenance. It has been linked to shorter stays in intensive care. Unfavorable side effects like nausea, colic, vomiting, and anorexia are sometimes linked to an early return to oral or enteral feeding. Careful preoperative planning and the development of a postoperative nutrition care plan can help maintain nutrition status throughout surgery. Before surgery, the patient and the surgeon should decide on the postoperative nutrition care plan.

Establishing enteral nutrition access after major gastrointestinal surgeries has become standard practice. In patients with moderate to severe preoperative malnutrition, facilitating early enteral feeding can enhance surgical results. The advantages of enteral access exceed the risks of problems connected to enteral access in individuals with documented preoperative malnutrition. In patients who are undernourished before surgery or who are expected to have poor oral intake for a longer period (7–14 days), the intraoperative installation of a gastrostomy or jejunostomy tube for enteral access should be seriously considered. Apart from strategizing for nutrition support before surgery, it is crucial to discuss returning to an oral diet. Significant postoperative morbidity following upper gastrointestinal surgical resection may include delayed gastric emptying, prolonged ileus, obstruction, gastroesophageal reflux, and post-gastrectomy syndrome. Malnutrition, weight loss, and an increase in mortality are possible outcomes when these problems manifest. Patients can take an active part in their recovery with the help of preoperative education that informs them about normal and abnormal postoperative events. A certified dietitian will now frequently provide nutrition instruction in a variety of locations, such as diabetes clinics. For instance, several insurance companies now mandate preoperative nutrition education from a certified dietitian due to the high rate of malnutrition among patients undergoing bariatric surgery. Less information is available regarding the benefit of dietary education for patients having gastrointestinal cancer surgery. Preoperative education about expectations and pain management has been shown in several trials to reduce anxiety, and pain, enhance outcomes, and boost satisfaction in patients. Patients with GI cancer who routinely receive PN during chemotherapy do not appear to have better results (Seo et al., 2016). Patients receiving adjuvant PN during chemotherapy do not have improvements in tumor response, bone marrow suppression, or patient survival. Though they should only be used for individuals for whom active treatment alternatives are still available and who are obviously malnourished and at risk of their malnutrition getting worse, PN, and EN do play a role in the primary treatment of malnutrition that may be perceived as a side effect of chemotherapy.

2.14. Immunonutrition

Numerous research studies have looked into the effects of immunonutrition which is EN supplemented with micro or macronutrients to maintain or enhance immune function and, in turn, improve outcomes for patients with GI cancer. Nucleic acids, omega-3 fatty acids, glutamine (GLN), arginine (ARG), and combinations of these nutrients have all been investigated as immunity-enhancing agents in gastrointestinal cancer patients. Immunonutrition used perioperatively in patients undergoing major GI cancer resections has been shown to improve outcomes. The prevalent amino acid in the human body, glutamine (GLN), serves as a vital substrate for cells that divide quickly, including lymphocytes, macrophages, enterocytes, fibroblasts, and the renal epithelium. The usefulness of enteral GLN alone has not been thoroughly studied, as it is frequently combined with other immunonutrients. Randomized research using parenteral GLN during surgery in patients with colorectal cancer found that glutamine supplementation improved the nitrogen balance. Essential for good health, the n-3 fatty acids promote the formation of leukotrienes in the 5-series and prostaglandins in the 3-series of PGE_3, which are linked to decreased inflammatory responses and enhanced immunocompetence (Shapiro et al., 1994). Weight stabilization can be achieved by taking n-3 fatty acid supplements in the range of 2–3 g daily. Leukotriene 5 levels rise and TNF levels fall in colon cancer patients receiving parenteral n-3 fatty acid supplementation. Research utilizing ARG in conjunction with additional immunonutrients demonstrates enhanced immunological characteristics and a reduced risk of infection in patients having cancer-related elective upper and lower gastrointestinal surgery. Compared to controls, patients with colorectal cancer who received preoperative parenteral ARG showed increased immune response.

Nucleotide supplementation had no effect on survival in patients with colorectal cancer. The term chemoprevention describes the use of drugs, vitamins, or other treatments to prevent cancer or its recurrence. Dietary components may have chemoprotective effects through a variety of mechanisms, such as cytochrome activation or inhibition, carcinogen detoxification, antioxidant activity, immune stimulation, physiology changes, and hormonal effects. All gastrointestinal diseases have obesity as a risk factor. It has been suggested to take many general dietary measures to prevent gastrointestinal cancer. A plant-based, low-fat diet combined with appropriate exercise and physical activity is one of these dietary adjustments. There seem to be chemopreventive effects of calcium and vitamin D in the colon and rectum. Colon epithelial hyperproliferation appears to be reduced by calcium, however vitamin D appears to moderate the effects of calcium. Secondary bile acids and ionized fatty acids are bound by calcium, which promotes the growth of the colorectal mucosal epithelial cells. Early research on the effect of calcium on the risk of colorectal cancer produced contradictory results. The gastrointestinal system is shielded by green tea. The main active ingredients in green tea that have been found to be chemoprotective are catechins, particularly EGCG (epigallocatechin gallate). Flavonols, caffeine, phenolic acid, thearubins, and taste compounds are some of the other ingredients in green tea. The GI tract's chemoprotective impact is thought to be caused by anticancer mechanisms such as *H.pylori* inhibition, chronic gastritis prevention, nitrosamine compound reduction, decreased carcinogen conversion, and altered gut microbiota.

A malabsorption syndrome brought on by significant intestinal resection is known as short bowel syndrome (SBS) (Figure 2.10). Necrotizing enterocolitis and congenital intestinal abnormalities are often the cause of intestinal problems in infants. The frequent causes of SBS in older children and adults are trauma, radiation enteritis, multiple resections for Crohn's disease, and major resections resulting from catastrophic mesenteric vascular events. Chronic diarrhea, dehydration, and deficits in macro and micronutrients are common in these patients, who frequently need home enteral or parenteral nutrition therapy. Nutrient absorption studies have shown that individuals who absorb less than 1.4 kg/day of wet weight, or less than 84% of their estimated energy requirements, are likely to need parenteral fluid and/or nutrition supplementation (Van Gossum et al., 2009). This usually corresponds to a patient having less than 50–70 cm of small bowel in the case of an intact colon or less than 100–150 cm in the case of an absent colon. SBS in adults is defined as having less than 200 centimeters of the residual small intestine. The length of the remaining colon, age, and the presence or absence of an ileocecal valve all affect how much resection is necessary to cause malabsorption in babies.

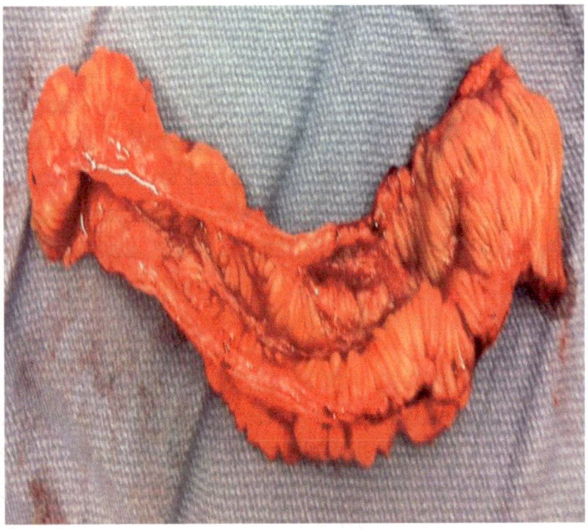

Figure 2.10. *Short bowel syndrome.*

Source: https://upload.wikimedia.org/wikipedia/commons/6/67/ResectedIleum.jpg, Creative Commons License.

Although SBS is rare, it nevertheless poses a significant clinical challenge because of the impact it has on the quality and length of life of these patients, the high frequency of related comorbidities, and the ensuing high costs of their treatment. It has been demonstrated that HPN patients, many of whom had SBS, had a lower quality of life than SBS patients who did not require PN. The end-jejunostomy and ultra-short small bowel groups had the lowest survival rates. The patient's age, the main disease process, any comorbid conditions, the existence of a chronic intestinal blockage, and the team's level of competence in handling the patient are other variables that impact survival. The ileum possesses tight intercellular connections than the jejunum. As a result, less sodium and water are moved. Concentrating the contents of the fluid and allowing for considerable reabsorption are made possible by sodium chloride active transport. The ileum is the site of production of numerous gastrointestinal (GI) hormones, including peptide YY and glucagon-like peptides 1 & 2, as well as the principal site of carrier-mediated bile salt and B_{12} absorption. The regulation of colon development and motility is aided by these GI hormones. Studies on individuals who have previously had ileocecal valve excision have not supported the earlier concept that the ileocecal valve helps to slow transit and prevent reflux of colonic contents into the small bowel. The retention of a large portion of the terminal ileum may be the reason for reports indicating a benefit associated with the ileocecal valve. When predicting the clinical prognosis of small bowel surgery patients, knowledge about the residual small bowel length can be helpful. However, it is frequently challenging to determine a precise measurement of bowel length. Although surgical reports are the best source of information, these notes often document the quantity of bowel removed rather than the quantity that is still there.

2.15. Research on Short Bowel Syndrome

The length, location, and presence of the colon are among the anatomical factors that influence the prognosis of patients with SBS (Massironi et al., 2020). While the jejunum primarily undergoes functional adaptation, the ileum can adapt both structurally and functionally, making jejunal resection generally more tolerable. Most SBS patients have had their ileum removed, leaving a section of the jejunum, often with part of the colon. For those with a jejuno-colic anastomosis, evidence supports functional adaptation of the small bowel. The colon plays a beneficial role in SBS by absorbing fatty acids, water, and electrolytes, slowing intestinal transit, and promoting intestinal adaptation. The presence of at least half of the colon is thought to be equivalent to approximately 50 cm of small bowel in terms of PN requirements. While most adult SBS patients with less than 50 cm of jejunum attached to the colon require long-term PN, patients with a jejuno-colic anastomosis and at least 100 cm of jejunum may not (Billiauws et al., 2018). Individuals without a colon and less than 100 cm of jejunum likely need lifelong PN. The colon, capable of absorbing up to 6 liters of fluid daily, is critical for fluid and electrolyte reabsorption, and its total loss often results in issues with electrolyte imbalances and dehydration in SBS patients. The proximal colon and ileum produce enteroglucagon, neurotensin, and peptide YY, which induce the jejunal, ileal, and colonic brake phenomena, slowing small intestine transit in response to fat intake. In addition to its absorptive capabilities, the colon hosts bacteria that convert malabsorbed carbohydrates into short-chain fatty acids, which are then absorbed, providing a significant energy source of up to 1,000 kcal per day.

There is no consensus on the significance of the oral diet in the management of SBS due to the limited experimental data about the role of luminal nutrients in human health. An optimum diet must be translated into foods and meal plans that fit the individual preferences, lifestyle, and, in the case of children, developmental stage for it to be successful over the long term. This involves intensive education and monitoring to ensure compliance. It is crucial to set daily targets for the patient's consumption of calories and fluids, followed by close monitoring and modifications based on tolerance as indicated by the emergence of symptoms, stool output, micronutrient levels, weight, and state of hydration. The computed resting energy expenditure multiplied by activity and malabsorption factors can generally be used to establish individual calorie needs. Since stable adult SBS patients only absorb half to two-thirds of what they normally would, food intake needs to be enhanced by at least 50%. It is usually recommended to consume a larger amount of food throughout the day in five to six meal periods. To meet their calorie needs, certain patients of any age may benefit from supplemental tube feeding, especially when attempting to wean PN. The majority of SBS patients with a colon can maintain adequate hydration without excessive fluid loss with hypotonic fluids, while those without a colon typically require the use of a glucose electrolyte oral rehydration solution (ORS) to enhance absorption and reduce secretion due to regional variations in water and sodium handling. However, ORS might still be helpful in the SBS with a colon, and the amount of sodium in the ORS might not need to be as high as long as the diet contains enough sodium.

Although the composition of the fluids is less significant in colon patients, they nevertheless need to consume enough salt in their diet. Hyperosmolar drinks, like ordinary soda and fruit juices, should be avoided regardless of the structure of the intestine, as they will exacerbate stool losses. Clinical experience indicates that individuals who frequently have bowel movements right after eating may benefit from refraining from drinking fluids during meals, even if there is not enough data to support this practice. If the ostomy output continues to surpass fluid intake, parenteral fluids will be required. It is recommended that people with SBS have complex macronutrients in their diet. In addition to lowering the osmotic burden, complex carbohydrates may aid in the adaptation process. Lactose is often well tolerated and should not be restricted unless the patient is clearly intolerant, as milk-based products are an important source of calories and calcium. This is because the proximal jejunum is rarely resected in individuals with SBS. Fruit juices in particular are concentrated sugars that should be avoided since they increase stool production and create a high osmotic load. High biological value proteins, such as those found in beef, pork, chicken, and fish, are preferable in terms of protein. It is advised that adult SBS patients with colons limit their daily calorie intake to 20% to 30% fat due to these causes (Matarese et al., 2005). As a result, there is less steatorrhea, less loss of calcium and magnesium, and less absorption of oxalate. In the absence of fat malabsorption, dietary oxalate is free to enter the colon, where it is absorbed and then filtered by the kidney. Normally, dietary oxalate binds to calcium and is eliminated in the stool. When oxalate binds to calcium in the kidney, it causes oxalate nephropathy. To reduce the risk of oxalate nephropathy, which can happen in up to 25% of SBS patients with a colon, oxalate limitation is crucial. To manage stool losses in SBS, antimotility, and antisecretory medicines are often needed on a long-term basis. Gastritis and gastric hypergastrinemia are temporary side effects of massive enterectomy. Proton pump inhibitors and H_2 receptor antagonists may help lower the volume of gastric secretions and consequently stool losses, especially in the first year after resection. The acidity may cause peptic issues and/or compromise the ability of the digestive enzymes to work. Acid-suppressing drugs should be used with caution *in situ*ations where there is bacterial overgrowth since gastric acid plays a part in reducing the growth of upper intestine bacteria. It is uncommon for certain people to benefit from treatment with octreotide, an analog of somatostatin, especially those who are net secretors like those who have high-output jejunostomies. Octreotide slows the transit of the jejunum and decreases the production of certain gastrointestinal secretions. Octreotide should only be used in patients with large volume stool losses in whom fluid and electrolyte management is problematic. It should also be avoided in the immediate period following intestinal resection due to the drug's increased risk of cholelithiasis, cost, and studies in animal models suggesting that it may inhibit bowel adaptation.

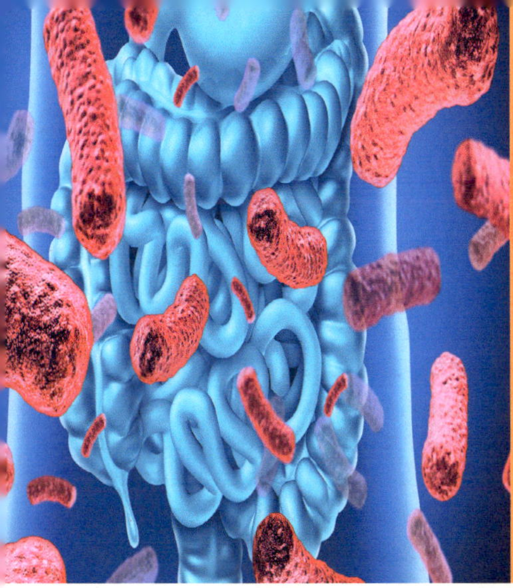

Chapter 3

PROBIOTICS AND GI HEALTH

Contents

3.1. Introduction

The diverse populations of microorganisms that reside on and within the human body are referred to as the human microbiome (Pflughoeft and Versalovic, 2012). The majority of these microorganisms are bacteria, but there are also viruses, fungi, archaea, and bacteriophages present. The human body has microbiomes in a variety of locations, such as the skin, mouth, nasopharynx, and genito-urinary tract. The genetic composition of the host as well as environmental factors, such as humidity, pH, nutrition, and oxygen levels influence the varying microbiome compositions. The human body depends on the microbiome for many vital processes, such as aiding in digestion and metabolism, generating vitamins, preserving the intestinal barrier, and controlling immune system development. Some research studies have linked microbiome dysbiosis to a higher risk of non-communicable diseases or NCDs, which include diabetes, obesity, asthma, and autoimmune disorders like Crohn's disease (Figure 3.1).

These conditions are due to an overactive immune system, which exacerbates pro-inflammatory status. The first 1000 days of life, or from conception to the first two years of life, are critical for the development and maturity of the immune system as well as for the colonization and establishment of pioneer microbes within the human body. Any disruptions to the gradual colonization of the new microbiota have the potential to increase short- and long-term risk of acquiring diseases. Recent scientific data, however, points to the possibility that the first microbial encounter occurs before birth and that it may even be crucial to fetal development.

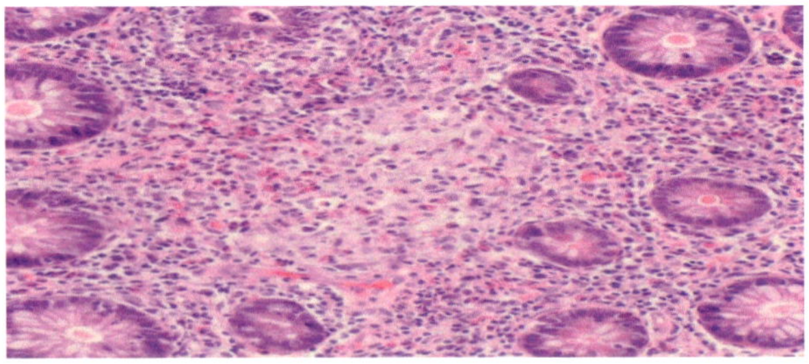

Figure 3.1. *Crohn's disease.*

Source: https://upload.wikimedia.org/wikipedia/commons/3/31/Histopathology_of_granuloma_of_colonic_mucosa.jpg, Creative Commons License.

3.2. Microbiota

Our understanding of the sterile environment and the early stages of microbiota colonization has changed as a result of several research studies. However, the prenatal and postnatal microbial source for the fetus and, eventually, the newborn is the mother's microbiota. However, the various prenatal variables that can impact the mother microbiota and, in turn, the fetal microbiota are still unclear despite the expanding relevant knowledge. More than 200 bacterial species make up the complex ecosystem known as the vaginal microbiota in healthy non-pregnant women. Lactobacillus species predominate, followed by less common species like Prevotella, Streptococcus, Bacteroides, and Veillonella. Different types of microbial communities that differ in terms of both composition and abundance have been described based on the Lactobacillus composition. These communities can be grouped into community state types (CSTs), each of which is home to a particular species of bacteria. The location (geographic) and ethnic origin of the individual affect the prevalence of the various CSTs. For instance, research in the USA has shown that African-American and Hispanic women have greater rates of CSTIV. The *Lactobacillus* genus is crucial for maintaining a low pH and secreting metabolites to stop pathogenic colonization in the vagina. An increasing amount of research has shown how the Lactobacillus species may be used as biomarkers of vaginal health. But the microbiota in the vagina does not stay constant. In fact, some researchers discovered that the vaginal microbiota exhibited temporal dynamics throughout two weeks, with certain communities changing and others remaining largely stable based on the CST. As little is currently known about the influence the vaginal microbiota has on the various bacterial populations or the short- and long-term effects on an individual's general health state, recent research has highlighted the necessity to analyze the host variables that affect the microbiota.

3.3. Infections and the Microbiome

There are microorganisms in the female reproductive system that affect women's health outside of the vagina. A specific endometrial microbiome found in the uterus has been related to reproductive and uterine health. High levels of *Lactobacillus, Prevotella, Atopobium*, and *Sneathia* have also been found in the vagina (endometrial microbiota) (Doroftei et al., 2023). The population of endometrial bacteria appears to differ somewhat from that of the vagina, indicating a connected but distinct relationship between the two microbiotas. It is known that bacteria from the genera *Pseudomonas, Staphylococcus, Enterococcus, Prevotella, and Propionibacterium* inhabit the fallopian tubes. The relationship between commensal bacteria in the uterus, fertility, and pregnancy difficulties has been highlighted by recent studies, which is significant. However, not much research has been done in the past on the male microbiota found in the reproductive system. Recent research has shown that semen contains microbiota. The most common phyla found in semen are the Firmicutes, which are followed by the Bacteroidetes, Actinobacteria, and Proteobacteria of which the most common genera are *Lactobacillus, Prevotella, Gillisia, Gardnerella, Corynebacterium.*

Male vaginal inflammatory issues have been linked to the prevalence of *Gardnerella vaginalis* (Figure 3.2) in the vaginal microbiome, which may be associated with vaginal colonization or infection. It has also been proposed that there is a connection between the reproductive microbiomes of men and women that affects health, gestation, reproduction, and fertility. Actually, previous studies on the semen microbiome have concentrated on the problem of infertility, revealing variations in the microbial diversity. Compared to healthy men, patients with obstructive or non-obstructive azoospermia had distinct seminal microbiomes, which revealed an increase in Bacteroidetes and Firmicutes and a decrease in Proteobacteria and Actinobacteria. When combined, the uterine and seminal microbiomes seem to be very important for reproductive medicine. Research points to the possibility that certain microbiota profiles could be used as biomarkers to help create novel techniques for the detection and management of infertility.

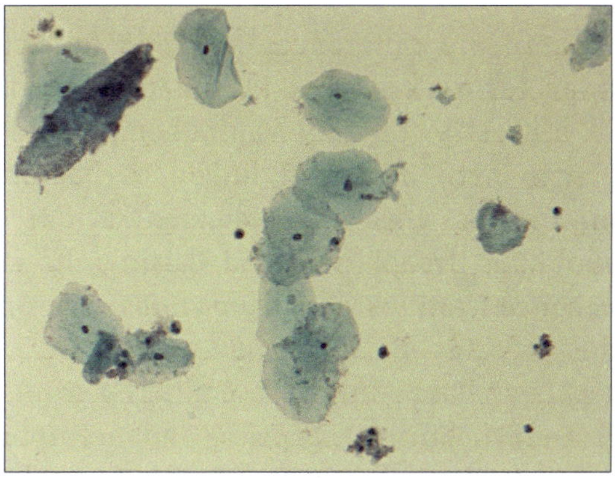

Figure 3.2. *Gardnerella vaginalis.*

Source: https://upload.wikimedia.org/wikipedia/commons/f/fb/G.vaginalis.jpg, Creative Commons License.

Since human reproduction occurs in a microbial environment, microorganisms need to be given more consideration because of their significance from conception onward. To provide the fetus with the best intrauterine environment and thus support proper growth, the mother's physiology and metabolism are altered throughout pregnancy. Maternal microbiota at various body sites, including as the vagina, stomach, and oral cavity, exhibits distinct variations that are indicative of gestational physiological changes, such as endocrine, immunological, and metabolic changes that favor a pro-inflammatory condition. While Lactobacillus species increase during pregnancy, likely strengthening their protective role, the vaginal microbiota microbial diversity diminishes. The fetus and infant may benefit from the uterine bacteria, which favor tolerance towards organisms that improve postnatal well-being, including the *Lactobacillus genus.* But there is growing evidence that dysbiosis in the vaginal microbiome during pregnancy increases the risk of premature delivery. The disturbances of this kind have been shown to happen as early as the first trimester. Further evidence suggests that women with a medical history of recurrent UTIs are more likely to give birth before full term.

There are differences between full-term and preterm deliveries in the composition and diversity of the vaginal microbiota. Preterm birth has been linked to bacterial communities with high concentrations of Atopobium, Ureaplasma, and Gardnerella and low concentrations of *Lactobacillus spp.* or a higher presence of *Candida albicans* (Figure 3.3). There is a chance that the seminal microbiota will disturb both conception and premature birth. Preterm births have been linked to high levels of common seminal bacteria, including *L. iners*, during pregnancy; in contrast, the predominance of *L. crispatus*, another common bacterial species in semen, is protective (Koort et al., 2023). The identification of anomalies in the vaginal microbiome during pregnancy may offer fresh perspectives on microbial indicators for anticipating the risk of an early birth.

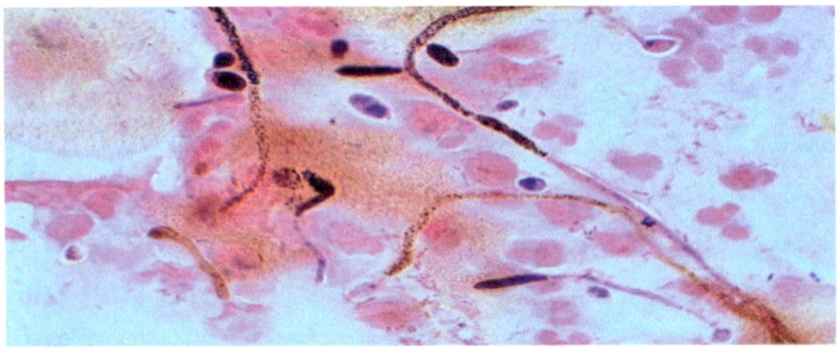

Figure 3.3. *Candida albicans.*

Source: https://upload.wikimedia.org/wikipedia/commons/e/e6/Candida_Gram_stain.jpg, Creative Commons License.

3.4. Gut Microbiota Dynamics

The composition of the gut microbiota changes intensely after the first trimester of pregnancy, while it stays stable and resembles the pre-pregnancy microbiome during this time. Some studies have shown that during pregnancy, the gut microbiota alters to reflect a more pro-inflammatory character, resembling alterations seen in cases of diabetes or metabolic syndrome. This inflammatory state is linked to metabolic adjustments throughout pregnancy and promotes a healthy pregnancy, which is advantageous for the growth of the fetus. The major alterations are characterized by a growth in the diversity of gut bacteria, a decrease in butyrate-producing bacteria, and an abundance of Proteobacteria and Actinobacteria. Research studies have not shown any appreciable microbial alterations in the gut during pregnancy, suggesting that more investigation is required to understand the effects of pregnancy on the gut microbiota. It has been extensively shown that exposure to antibiotics during pregnancy modifies the bacterial environment, which in turn affects the microbiome. Pregnancy-related antibiotic use increases the Staphylococcus colonization of the vagina, and possible microbial changes in places other than the gut may increase the risk of allergies and obesity. The mother's nutritional state and food have an impact on the maternal microbiome during pregnancy. According to recent reports, the mother's diet during pregnancy has a significant effect on the microbiotas of the mother and the unborn child. The pre-gestational body mass index (BMI) of the mother and weight growth during pregnancy may have an impact on the changes in the female gut microbiota. When compared to lean mothers who maintained a weight gain following recommendations, there was a lower presence of *Bifidobacterium* spp. in overweight and obese mothers, as well as in mothers who gained excessive weight during pregnancy. Similar changes in weight status throughout pregnancy were also noted in some studies. Overweight pregnant women were shown to have abundances of Staphylococcus species and *Escherichia coli*, and lower levels of *Bacteroides* spp. Such alterations in the mother gut microbiota may be linked to variations in the process of intestinal colonization in newborns delivered via the vagina.

3.5. Oral Microbiome

The oral microbiome is altered during pregnancy. When comparing the loads of several species in the oral cavities of pregnant and non-pregnant women, prominent changes have been documented. Increases in the numbers of viable bacteria and higher concentrations of pathogenic bacteria, such as Actinomycetemcomitans, *Aggregatibacter actinomycetemcomitans* (Figure 3.4), *Porphyromonas gingivalis*, and Candida, are characteristics of the oral microbiota during pregnancy (Saadaoui et al., 2021).

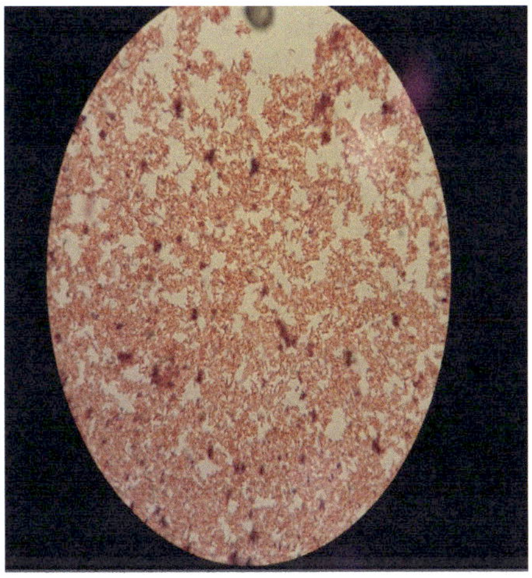

Figure 3.4. *Aggregatibacter actinomycetemcomitans.*

Source: https://upload.wikimedia.org/wikipedia/commons/5/54/The_Gram_Staining_-_Bacteria_Gram_Negative.JPG, Creative Commons License.

These findings support the research linking periodontal disease and oral infections to pregnancy complications, including preterm delivery. These findings imply that the oral microbiota is also important for maternal and neonatal outcomes, such as early microbial colonization in the fetus and neonatal stages, pregnancy problems, and preterm delivery risk. To minimize undesirable microbial alterations during pregnancy, which may be connected to pregnancy problems, more research on the relationship between microbial indicators and pregnancy outcomes may be very helpful. The human microbiota has been studied in previously considered sterile areas, such as the placenta, meconium, and fetal membranes. Bacteria from those regions have been isolated and identified in certain investigations. Despite several studies in the field, it is still unclear if the presence of microorganisms in these locations would indicate the presence of a particular microbiota niche (placenta microbiota) and what their biological significance would be. There is no proof of early microbial contact or a placenta microbiome. The low quantity of DNA and potential bias resulting from contaminating DNA, as well as its detection raises the likelihood of false positive results, are the crucial problems.

The debated theory proposes either a hematogenous route or a vertical ascendant route from the vagina to the fetus. It is important to remember that recent research has indicated that healthy people may have a blood microbiome. It has been documented that the presence of placenta-derived exosomes and fetal DNA in the maternal circulation may indicate a possible link between these substances and preterm birth risk, placenta health, and preeclampsia. Previous research on the placental microbiome has postulated that the primary source of the bacteria found in placenta tissue may be the oral microbiota. There is evidence to suggest that the composition of the placental microbiome may have a stronger correlation with the oral microbiota than with the vaginal or gut microbiota. These findings are corroborated by the link that has been shown between problematic pregnancy outcomes, including premature birth, and inflammatory oral disease, primarily periodontitis. In the placental microbiome of preterm patients with chorioamnionitis, some researchers found a progressive increase in oral commensal bacteria. This shows the significance of *Fusobacterium nucleatum*, a common oral bacterium found in the placenta, concerning unfavorable pregnancy outcomes, such as preterm birth, neonatal sepsis, and hypertension. Animal models have been used to demonstrate the oral-fetoplacental pathway. However, it has been shown in animal models that during pregnancy, there is an increase in microbial translocation from the gastrointestinal (GI) tract. The intricate relationships between bacteria and the immune system, which are in turn mediated by the GI tract dendritic cells, may be responsible for this translocation. Orally administered *Enterococcus faecium* was discovered in both the placenta tissue and meconium (Li et al., 2021).

3.6. Fetal Microbiota

Since the fetus continuously swallows amniotic fluid, it establishes contact with the fetal gut throughout gestation, making it particularly significant for researching the impact of the microbiota on neonatal health. A bacterium found in amniotic fluid is considered to be indicative of a health problem since it can lead to chorioamnionitis, an infection of the amniotic cavity that accounts for 25% of preterm births. Due to the link between preterm birth and amniotic fluid bacteria, research on the amniotic fluid microbiome in these situations may be crucial to preventing preterm birth or even elucidating potential molecular pathways through which particular bacterial populations may adversely affect a pregnancy course. The amniotic fluid of preterm mothers has previously been reported to include a distinct microbial population, with Ureaplasma and Mycoplasma species being prominent. Some researchers found that children with severe chorioamnionitis and preterm mothers with the same disease had distinct placental microbiomes, with Fusobacterium and Ureaplasma predominating in this instance. Studies have shown bacterial DNA in the amniotic fluid of healthy mothers. However, the theory about the existence of bacteria in healthy people's amniotic cavities is still up for debate, in part because of inconsistent findings. Studies have also revealed that the amniotic fluid contains no bacteria. Some researchers revealed that bacterial DNA loads in the amniotic fluid originating from intact membranes were similar to those observed in negative controls. Anaerobic culturing could only be carried out in amniotic fluid derived from ruptured membranes. Researchers discovered bacterial DNA in the amniotic fluid taken from healthy, term pregnancies without clinical infection symptoms. The microbial populations identified in healthy amniotic fluid are primarily Proteobacteria, particularly those belonging to the Enterobacter and Shigella genera, as well as Propionibacterium species, and they should be highly comparable to those seen in the placenta.

3.7. Investigative Findings and Theories

Systematic investigations regarding the significance of the pregnancy period to the colonization process have been made possible by the suggestion made by certain researchers that there is bacterial DNA in the placenta and amniotic fluid. This suggests that the colonization process may have started in utero. Some research indicates the presence of bacteria in the meconium, the first newborn stool that represents life in utero, as determined by culture-dependent and culture-independent techniques. This suggests microbial colonization before birth. Nonetheless, other researchers have proposed that the presence of bacteria in the meconium could be explained by the possibility that neonatal colonization begins during uterine contraction and membrane rupture. The babies delivered by elective cesarean section and non-elective cesarean section had meconium microbiota profiles that were similar. The *Proteobacteria* and *Firmicutes phyla*, including the Enterobacteriaceae and Enterococcaceae families, comprise the meconium microbiota (Lee et al., 2020). These bacteria are typically more prevalent in the microbiota in adulthood than in infancy, indicating their maternal origin.

Other genera were discovered, such as Bifidobacterium, Bacteroides, and Prevotella. Compared to the oral or maternal vaginal microbiota, the meconium microbiota has been found to have higher similarities with the amniotic fluid, which may be related to the meconium bacterial origins. The bacteria that are shared by the placenta and the fetal intestine have also been reported in recent animal research studies. Many maternal factors, such as diabetes, atopic dermatitis, maternal diet, BMI, and perinatal antibiotic use, have been linked to changes in the meconium microbiota. Scientists found that the meconium of infants born to mothers with pregestational type 2 diabetes mellitus included an enrichment of bacteria typically found in adult diabetic patients. A high-fat maternal diet affects the meconium microbiota, causing a noticeable reduction of the Bacteroides genus.

In the first week of life, some researchers demonstrated that the administration of intrapartum antibiotics could change the intestinal microbiota, resulting in a decrease in Actinobacteria and a progressive increase in Proteobacteria and Firmicutes loads. Antibiotics given during childbirth may similarly alter the oral microbiome in newborns, leading to an increase in the number of *Proteobacteria phylum* species after the antibiotic treatment. Researchers found that there was an 84% increased risk of obesity development among children exposed to antibiotic treatment throughout the second and third trimesters of pregnancy. It is presently unknown how they might affect the immune system, metabolism, and overall health.

Although there is increasing evidence regarding the immunomodulatory activity of the gut microbiota in both disease and health during childhood and adulthood, the molecular mechanisms by which the placenta, meconium microbiota, and amniotic fluid affect immune system development remain incompletely understood. Metabolites (microbial) in the fetal environment can have a significant effect on the development of the immune system and newborn development. It is known that metabolites and byproducts of microbes can enter the bloodstream and migrate to many sites.

As a result, metabolites originating from the maternal microbiota may cross the placenta and end up in the amniotic fluid and breast milk. These findings highlight the possible influence of microorganisms and their byproducts on the developing fetus and point to the necessity of expanding our understanding to support fetal health. Mothers can transmit bacteria vertically to their offspring.

In addition to bacteria from the environment, the newborn also comes into contact with a vast array of germs from the mother's stomach and vagina during delivery. A delicate, dynamic, step-by-step process that is especially pertinent to health is newborn colonization. Premature birth, the method of delivery, and early nursing practices are among the maternal and newborn variables that may have an impact on the process. Low microbial diversity and richness and a comparatively larger abundance of Proteobacteria and Actinobacteria phyla define the gut microbiota of newborns (Rinninella et al., 2019).

3.8. Vaginal Microbiome and Breastmilk

Previous research studies have shown that newborns delivered via the vagina have a microbiota that resembles the vaginal microbiome, enriched with Lactobacillus and Prevotella species, though other bacteria, such as those from the Enterobacteriaceae family, which includes Escherichia or Klebsiella, are also present. Cesarean section babies had unique microbiota that resembled the oral, cutaneous, and ambient microbiota that is dominated by Propionibacterium, Corynebacterium, and Staphylococcus. Since 72% of the gut bacteria in neonates delivered vaginally are of maternal intestinal origin, compared to 41% in subjects born via cesarean section, the mother's gut also seems to be a significant source of early colonizing bacteria. Children delivered by cesarean section showed lower diversity and delayed colonization of the Bacteroides genus. Breastmilk promotes immune system maturation and aids in the microbial colonization of the newborn gut. There have been reports of differences in the newborn microbiota between formula-fed and breastfed infants. However, recent research has indicated that the introduction of solid and complementary foods, rather than the discontinuation of breastfeeding, had a significant effect on the infant microbiome. Although research studies have revealed the presence of Staphylococcus, Streptococcus, and certain Proteobacteria in breast milk samples, human milk has always been thought to be sterile. It has also been common to identify and isolate Lactobacillus and Bifidobacterium. The infant's gut gets 27.7% of its bacteria from breast milk and 10.3% from the skin of the areola. This finding raises questions about the possible effects of breastfeeding on the child's gut microbiota. It has been determined that breast milk and the developing baby gut share certain microbial and viral species. Numerous other factors have also been extensively researched that include antibiotics, gestational age, other environmental factors, and host genetics, including geographic location, rural areas, siblings, pet ownership, etc. It has been demonstrated that these elements, either separately or in combination, affect the development of the immune system and microbiota. The neonatal intensive care units (NICUs) are populated with infants suffering from the necrotizing enterocolitis (NEC) (Ergenekon et al., 2021). NEC is characterized by ischemic bowel necrosis and has long been associated with microbial dysbiosis in preterm newborns. Research on NEC risk factors is ongoing in an effort to create better preventative and therapeutic interventions. Considering the microbiome's contribution to NEC pathogenesis, it seems like a promising target for treatment. All microorganisms that live in the human mouth, skin, stomach, and urogenital tract and human somatic cells making up less than 1% of the body mass on average are collectively referred to as the human microbiota. Thousands of distinct bacterial species can be found in the microbial community, and they are essential to preserving homeostasis, which includes the growth and maintenance of several organ systems, including the gut, endocrine system, lungs, bone, liver, and brain. Around the time of birth, microbial colonization starts, and by the time a toddler reaches the age of three, their diet starts to resemble that of their adult counterparts. Early-life dysbiosis, or a change toward a pathogenic imbalance of microorganisms, has been linked to a variety of disease states, such as type I diabetes, autoimmune disorders, food allergies, and obesity.

3.9. Feeding Practices and Antibiotics

Since the microbiome can usually be changed

quickly, it offers a unique target for therapy. One method of influencing the microbiome to enhance health outcomes is the direct delivery of probiotics, which are live organisms that benefit the host. Other possible strategies for changing microbiota include limiting the use of preventative antibiotics, fecal transplantation, and prebiotic supplementation. Another interesting therapeutic target for newborns is the modification of the mother microbiota during pregnancy and lactation. During delivery and shortly after, the microbes (maternal and environmental) start to rapidly colonize the infant's intestinal tract. Early microbial colonization is caused by a variety of factors, such as feeding practices, environmental factors, early antibiotic usage, delivery mode-dependent vertical transmission during birth, and possibly even intrauterine transmission. Early colonization patterns have repeatedly been observed to be influenced by the mode of delivery. During pregnancy, the vaginal microbiome changes to favor Lactobacillus species, which may offer protection against harmful bacteria by keeping the pH low. The infants born vaginally are more easily colonized by their mother's vaginal microbiota, whereas infants delivered by cesarean section have microbiomes that most closely resemble bacteria found on their mother's skin in the early stages of life. It was discovered that in the first year of life, infants born via cesarean section shared less gut microbiota with their mothers and had a significantly lower variety of Bacteroides species than the majority of kids delivered vaginally. Diet and feeding practices have a variety of effects on the formation of the microbiome. Compared to infants who are exclusively breastfed, formula-fed infants have been reported to have less desirable bacteria species, such as *Clostridium difficile* (Figure 3.5) (Inchingolo et al., 2024). As a result of interaction with the areolar skin and the contents of breast milk, breastfeeding encourages the formation of a microbiome that more closely resembles that of the mother. Several genera of bacteria are shared by human breast milk and newborn fecal samples, with up to 70–88% of these genera being present. The vertical transmission of microbiota through nursing may also be influenced by the diet of the mother. The variations in the infant and mother diets were the cause of the differences observed between South Asian and Caucasian infant cohorts at one year of age. South Asians showed a higher abundance of Lactobacillales, while Caucasians showed a higher abundance of Clostridiales. Antibiotic therapy and environmental variables are also important in the early stages of colonization. Having more older siblings living at home is associated with higher neonatal microbial diversity, particularly from the phylum Firmicutes and Bacteroidetes. Infants receiving antibiotic treatment had lower bacterial diversity in terms of both species and strains.

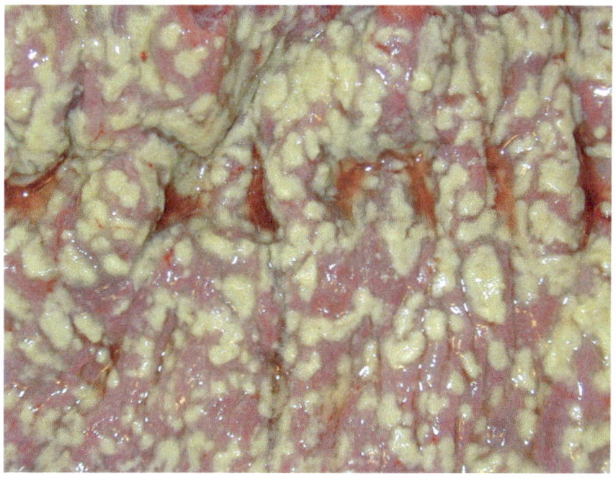

Figure 3.5. *Clostridium difficile.*

Source: https://upload.wikimedia.org/wikipedia/commons/a/a1/Pseudomembranous_colitis.JPG, Creative Commons License.

Antibiotic use by mothers before giving birth has also been linked to a decline in the variety of the infant microbiota, particularly in the absence of Bifidobacterium species, a genus that is typically thought to be advantageous. Even among healthy baby microbiomes, there is a lot of variance, but high levels of diversity are often seen as protective because they inhibit the proliferation of any one dominating organism. When unfavorable bacteria take over and raise the risk of disease, it is known as dysbiosis. Numerous kinds of bacteria have been linked to a wide range of diseases. The development of appropriate anatomical structures and physiological responses like immunologic, metabolic, and neurologic, has been linked to early microbial colonization. A higher chance of allergies later in life is linked to decreased Lactobacillus and *Bifidobacterium* spp. colonization during infancy. Childhood obesity has been linked to lower levels of *Bifidobacterium* spp. and higher levels of *Staphylococcus aureus* in early life. Concomitant microbiota is essential for healthy brain development as well. Studies using gnotobiotic mice have revealed that changes in the microbiota cause changes in the expression of insulin-like growth factor 1 (IGF-1), which is linked to perinatal growth. Poor development and cognitive impairment are linked to low IGF-1 levels.

3.10. Microbial Diversity in Preterm Infants

Compared to age-matched full-term infants, preterm, and low birth weight (LBW) babies show reduced microbial diversity across several body sites. Preterm baby skin, mouth, and gut were colonized by the same initial bacterial populations. This finding suggests that site overlap leads to a reduction in total diversity. This lack of diversity might make it easier for harmful organisms to proliferate and create the conditions necessary for disease. The variables such as delivery mode, feeding technique, and antibiotic use that are known to affect early colonization are also contributing factors to decreased diversity and dysbiosis in preterm infants. The mother's vaginal microbiome is another element influencing the microbiome of the preterm infant. Reduced microbial diversity during pregnancy has been linked to premature birth. Preterm babies may not have the same exposure to a rich vaginal microbiome as their term counterparts, even if they are delivered vaginally. Since the majority of preterm babies will spend their starting days in the neonatal intensive care unit or NICU, it is critical to look at the particular environmental conditions that lead to dysbiosis. For instance, it has been discovered that surfaces often used by newborns in the intensive care unit (NICU), such as ventilators, positive pressure airway machines, and incubators contain communities of Streptococcus, Staphylococcus, Neisseria, and Enterobacteriaceae. There is evidence that these colonies act as reservoirs for newborn gut colonization, which increases the risk of nosocomial infections and early dysbiosis. Typical NICU treatments might also be a factor in early dysbiosis (Parkin et al., 2021). Research studies showed that while treatment with antibiotics correlated with decreased abundance of Firmicutes and increased abundance of Proteobacteria, treatment with histamine receptor blockers (H2-blockers) or proton pump inhibitors (PPI), both of which act to reduce production of gastric acid, correlated with increased abundance of Proteobacteria, Actinobacteria, and Bacteroidetes. Necrotizing enterocolitis is characterized by ischemia of the gastrointestinal (GI) tract, followed by intestinal necrosis and the distinctive pneumatosis intestinalalis. Premature babies are the main victims of NEC, which first manifests as a swollen abdomen and nonspecific symptoms. There are three stages in NEC. The first stage, known as the suspect stage, is distinguished by GI symptoms and radiograph-visible abdominal distension. The definite stage II is characterized by several radiographic abnormalities such as edema, ileus, substantial intestinal distention, pneumatosis intestinalis, and portal vein gas in addition to GI bleeding. Stage III is the most advanced phase of the disease, characterized by intestinal necrosis, septic shock, gastrointestinal bleeding, and pneumoperitoneum on radiographs. Necrotic intestinal excision is necessary in stage III and necessitates surgical intervention. NEC affects up to 13% of preterm neonates in developed countries and has been growing with time. This trend is probably due to the rising survival rate of extremely preterm infants.

3.11. Neonate Cohort Studies

Neonates with bacterial infections and delivered by cesarean section have high rates of NEC. Higher rates of NEC are also linked to chromosomal abnormalities, cardiac malformations, and GI abnormalities. Furthermore, H2-blocker treatment is positively correlated with the occurrence of NEC (Iijima, 2024). It was discovered that breast milk consumption by premature newborns protects against NEC, with a dose-related decrease in the risk of developing NEC. Lack of bacterial diversity is a contributing factor to the development of NEC, which is consistent with these risks and protective factors. While all preterm infants show low overall diversity, some studies that looked at microbiome diversity using the Shannon diversity index discovered that preterm neonates who went on to develop NEC had lower diversity scores than their healthy preterm counterparts. It was discovered that the predominant Gammaproteobacteria genera in each of the newborns in the NEC group accounted for more than 50% of their bacterial colonization. It was discovered that the healthy controls did not exhibit this. When analyzing potential causes, it was shown that infants in the NEC group had received more days of antibiotic medication before having NEC, which probably helped explain why there was less variety in the NEC group compared to the control group. According to a different multisite, retrospective cohort analysis, the likelihood of developing NEC rose with every extra day of antibiotic treatment and there was a correlation between extended antibiotic therapy and NEC. The concept that lower microbial diversity increases the risk of pathogenic colonization and NEC in infants is supported by these datasets. Although some researchers suggest that live bacteria are necessary for the development of NEC, consistent isolation of particular species has not been achieved. Despite this, several species, mostly belonging to the phyla Firmicutes and Proteobacteria, have been linked to NEC; nevertheless, the mentioned microbes are also present in healthy newborns. The relative abundance and development of a single dominant species seem to be the fundamental difference in determining pathogenicity.

3.12. Bacterial Abundance in NEC

Many supporting studies have discovered that infants with NEC have higher relative abundances of Proteobacteria in their stool; however, some studies specifically report higher abundances of Gammaproteobacteria, including *Escherichia coli*, *Klebsiella* sp., and *Cronobacter sakazakii*. Coagulase-negative staphylococci (CoNS) belong to the phylum Firmicutes and are frequently detected in the feces of newborns diagnosed with NEC. Further, CoNS may benefit from the decreased function of the intestinal barrier resulting from parenteral nourishment. Despite being a component of the commensal microbiome of preterm neonates, *Clostridium* spp. and related toxins are also frequently found in large quantities in the stool of neonates with NEC and have been linked to severe outcomes and a faster progression of NEC. It is important to note that other nonbacterial organisms, like virus-associated NEC and Candida, may also be involved in the development of NEC in both protective and pathogenic ways. It is uncertain that a single pathogen will be identified as the only cause of NEC given the vast array of bacteria and diverse range of data gathered from many investigations. Knowing the components of the microbiome that could support the development of the host immune system and offer defense against NEC and other diseases is more crucial. Changing a preterm infant microbiome to promote healthy diversity may avoid NEC if microbial dysbiosis is, at least partially responsible for the development of NEC. Giving probiotics to preterm babies as a preventative measure to guard against NEC is undoubtedly a promising field of research. Randomized control trials (RCT) were compared to examine the efficacy of single-strain versus multi-strain probiotics (McFarland, 2021). Some researchers discovered that multi-strain probiotics significantly decreased the incidence of NEC, but single-strain probiotics showed either marginal benefits (Lactobacillus species) or no benefits at all (Bifidobacterium species) in lowering NEC or mortality. It is not unexpected that single-strain probiotics were not shown to impart any benefit, given they do not promote microbiome diversity.

3.13. The Promise of Probiotics

There may be some advantages to single-strain probiotic therapy. Rats fed with *Bifidobacterium adolescentis* showed higher survival rates and lower intestinal damage from NEC in a newborn rat model with induced NEC, indicating a preventive effect. The probiotic treatment increased the expression of single Ig IL-1-related receptor (SIGIRR) and toll-interacting protein (TOLLIP), which are responsible for moderating inflammation and maintaining homeostasis in the colonic epithelium, respectively, and decreased the expression of toll-like receptor 4 (TLR4). Even though there is evidence that probiotic therapy can lower the incidence of NEC, more clinical research needs to be done before recommendations can be made. The medical evidence for these beneficial effects is still lacking, despite the fact that many RCTs and cohort studies have been conducted to observe the impact of probiotic supplementation on the rate of NEC. Probiotic administration carries some concerns for premature and very low birth weight (VLBW) newborns. The risk of infections and sepsis, the variability of probiotics from different species and strains, and the absence of FDA or other agency regulation to guarantee the efficacy and safety of commercial products are some of the main issues surrounding the prophylactic administration of probiotics. The immune systems of premature and VLBW babies are underdeveloped. This is caused by a number of mechanisms, such as a decrease in complement protein, fewer circulating maternal IgG, and a decrease in neutrophils and monocytes. These deficits make it easier for even beneficial bacteria to proliferate, raising the possibility of infection and sepsis.

Probiotics should be given with caution to premature and VLBW newborns since they may not have the immune systems necessary to keep even commensal bacteria in control. The advantages and hazards of giving medication to a premature baby can vary depending on the distinct bioactivity exhibited by each strain or combination of strains. Natural variation may exist even among the same strain which could affect the consequences for infants. This poses a problem for consistency in manufacturing and regulation. It is unclear from a regulatory perspective whether probiotics should be regarded as food, dietary supplements, or medications (drugs). It makes sense for healthy people to consume probiotics as food. Probiotics are mostly consumed by most people through fermented foods, frequently without their awareness. Therefore, the majority of probiotics are sold as dietary supplements, subject to FDA regulation. The FDA only mandates that studies be done on healthy population subgroups to regulate health claims made for dietary supplements. However, there is a clear need for more investigation when probiotics are used to treat or prevent disease in susceptible populations, such as premature newborns. A preterm baby passed away in 2014 from a rare fungal infection called mucormycosis, which usually affects people with impaired immune systems. The newborn received a probiotic dietary supplement in the hospital that turned out to be contaminated with *Rhizopus oryzae*, which was the source of the infection. It is also important to note that not many research studies have looked into the long-term consequences of probiotic supplementation in newborns. Probiotics may have permanent effects on the immune system, metabolism, GI tract, and brain development if given at such a young age. More long-term trials that monitor newborns throughout childhood and adolescence are crucial to determine the therapy's safety as well as its long-term effects, even though they may be assumed to be positive.

Probiotics are a promising treatment with potential wide-ranging uses in medicine, but more stringent regulation and testing are required to guarantee the safety of vulnerable populations. To prevent NEC in NICU patients, only probiotics that have passed FDA medication testing and approval for the specific demographic should be utilized. Probiotics that are presently controlled as dietary supplements ought to be taken by people in good health only. This will assist in assuring the effectiveness and safety of probiotic administration among susceptible patients in NICUs. Probiotics given directly to premature infants is not the only therapeutic approach available to modify the early microbiome (Mercer and Arrieta, 2023). Prebiotics are indigestible dietary additives used to promote the growth of commensal microorganisms. In the case of humans, these are often prebiotics that are oligosaccharides, including fructooligosaccharides (FOS) and galactooligosaccharides (GOS). Prebiotics can be added to baby food formula to encourage the growth of Bifidobacterium and Lactobacillus. Prebiotics appear to be a viable therapy and preventive measure for infant colic. Prebiotic supplementation in preterm infants has been shown to change the fecal microbiota and have some benefits, however, some researchers found insufficient data to imply that prebiotics lower the incidence of NEC in human trials. It is also important to note that prebiotic supplements carry the same risk of contamination as probiotics, necessitating testing and regulation comparable to that of probiotics to protect the susceptible preterm population.

Human milk oligosaccharides (HMOs) are found in human breast milk, and they have a prebiotic role (Okburan and Kızıler, 2023). They also influence the microbial community of breastfed children. Preterm babies may receive less benefit from their mother's breast milk than those of mothers who give birth at term because of these differences. Certain HMOs that may provide protection against NEC have been identified through animal-based investigations. Reducing the use of antibiotics in NICUs is another possible strategy for influencing the preterm infant microbiome toward healthy microbial diversity. It is well-recognized that early antibiotic therapy for preterm infants reduces the diversity of gut microorganisms and causes dysbiosis. However, given any significant risk factor, such as an early rupture of the membranes or a maternal fever, doctors are required to prescribe prophylactic antibiotics to prevent infection to reduce the risk of newborn sepsis, a potentially fatal disease. To create standards for antibiotic use in NICUs, additional research and data are needed to balance the risks of suspected sepsis against antibiotic-related side effects. Modifying the mother's microbiome offers a possible way to modify the microbiome of the infant. It was discovered that the pups produced by manipulating the microbiome of pregnant mice through gastric gavage with human fecal homogenate shared the same microbial profile. There are several approaches to altering the microbiome during pregnancy to take into account, including supplementing with probiotics and prebiotics. Prebiotics FOS and GOS have been shown to boost maternal *Bifidobacterium* spp. when taken during pregnancy; however, the baby does not always benefit from this effect. It has been discovered that mothers benefit from prenatal probiotic consumption, which may have a protective effect against gestational diabetes, vaginal infections, and preeclampsia. Probiotics given during pregnancy, however, may lessen the likelihood that the fetus will develop eczema, rhinoconjunctivitis, and atopic dermatitis. Although probiotics intended for prenatal administration still need to be better regulated, the risks are lower when given to the mother than to a preterm child because of the mother's immune system maturation.

It is crucial to keep looking at alternatives to giving probiotics directly to preterm babies because there are many therapeutic targets for changing the microbiome of these babies. There is potential for avoiding and enhancing NEC outcomes with prebiotic supplements, breastfeeding, and changing the maternal microbial ecology. The majority of preterm babies are affected with necrotizing enterocolitis (NEC), which affects 7–10% of children with very low birth weight between the ages of 2 weeks and 2 months (Dilli et al, 2012). Its prevalence is inversely correlated with gestational age. The survivors (babies) are more likely to experience severe health issues like SBS and neurological problems. It is linked to a mortality rate of up to 30%. NEC has a significant financial cost, costing the US economy up to $1 billion a year. There is consensus regarding the multifactorial pathophysiology of the disease, which is caused by several overlapping risk factors, stresses, and/or acute intestine injury and inflammation. However, the precise biology of the disease is still not entirely understood. Therefore, the development of innovative preventative drugs is necessary. Microbiological diversity is low in preterm infants, and there is a higher chance of pathogenic colonization. Some reports have suggested that there might be a gestational threshold for the colonization of anaerobic and Bifidobacterium species, which are primarily represented from 33 weeks of gestation. Since no particular microbial pathogen has been identified as the etiologic agent responsible for the growth of the disease, data suggest that dysbiosis, particularly an increased concentration of Gram-negative facultative bacteria and a decrease in obligate anaerobes, may play a critical role in the pathogenesis of NEC. Preterm infants have an increased susceptibility to NEC development because the intestinal barrier, which guards against potentially harmful organisms, is still developing in these patients. This barrier is made up of several components, including the mucus coating, a layer of enterocytes tightly connected by a system of intracellular and membrane-spanning proteins, and an associated immune cells network.

3.14. Immune System Aspects

Numerous studies have highlighted the function that immune cells play in this context; more specifically, when NEC develops, an immune cell imbalance occurs that exacerbates the pro-inflammatory condition. The development of intestinal homeostasis is encouraged by intestinal regulatory T cells (Tregs), which are present from the 23rd week of pregnancy onward and are crucial in downregulating the pro-inflammatory response. The experimental models have shown that NEC development is characterized by a decrease in Tregs and an increase in Th17, which are linked to intestinal damage and increased enterocyte death (De Fazio et al., 2021).

Immune cells (*Lamina propria*) (Figure 3.6) and intestinal epithelial cells carry toll-like receptors

(TLRs), which play a major role in regulating the production of epithelial cells, the synthesis of IgA, the preservation of cell junctions, and the expression of antimicrobial peptides. TLR4 function in the pathophysiology of NEC has been extensively studied. TLR4 identifies lipopolysaccharides and triggers nuclear factor-κB, which initiates a chain reaction that promotes inflammation. The enterocyte death is promoted while intestinal epithelium repair is inhibited.

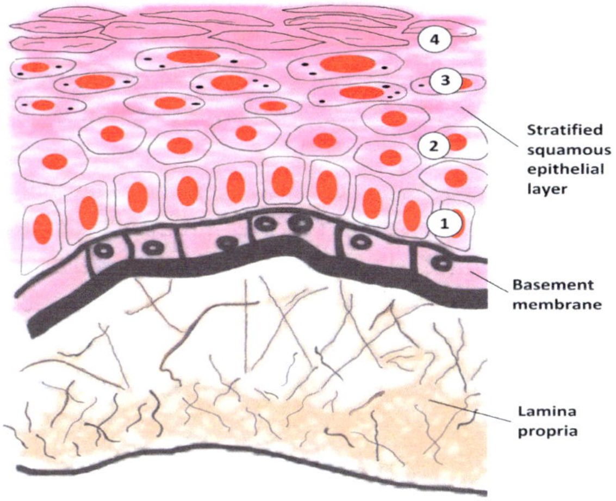

Figure 3.6. *Lamina propria.*

Source: https://en.wikipedia.org/wiki/Lamina_propria#/media/File:Oral_mucosa.png, Creative Commons License.

Therefore, mucosal damage and bacterial translocation into the bloodstream are caused by TLR4-mediated bacterial signaling. The interaction of bacteria and TRL4 on the lining of the mesenteric blood vessels results in a decrease in nitric oxide generation, severe vasoconstriction, and lower intestinal perfusion. Premature infants express TLR4 at significant levels. TLR4 signaling in intestinal epithelial cells throughout the early stages of life promotes tolerance development, which eases bacterial colonization and reduces inflammatory response. It is more challenging to achieve this control in premature infants. While breastfeeding has a dose-dependent protective effect, formula feeding has also been linked to a greater risk of NEC, with a risk ratio of 2.77. It has been proposed that formula feeding may play a role in the proliferation of bacteria and mucosal translocation that affect preterm infant gut microbiota. From early clinical manifestation to severe intestinal necrosis requiring surgical intervention and necrotic bowel resection, NEC progresses quickly. As a result, the efficacy of potential treatments is restricted to supportive care at the time of diagnosis, while research efforts have been directed at identifying NEC preventive approaches.

The successful approach to preventing NECs has been to promote breastfeeding. The precise processes behind human milk protective properties remain to be fully understood, but they involve the provision of immunoglobulins, growth factors like heparin-binding epidermal growth factor (EGF) and its metabolites, L-arginine, lactoferrin, oligosaccharides, nitrate/nitrite, and L-glutamine. The microorganisms are transferred to infants through the entero-mammary pathway in human milk, which further shapes the infant's immune system and microbiota. Probiotic administration has been suggested as a prophylactic measure to reduce preterm infant risk of necrotizing enterocolitis. The probiotics are live microorganisms that, when consumed in sufficient quantities, boost the host's health. This definition also applies to commensal bacteria. However, recent research suggests that not all of the benefits to health are directly connected to bacterial survival. A postbiotic is any soluble component produced by the metabolic activity of live bacteria or any released chemical that has the potential to improve health via a direct or indirect mechanism. Compared to probiotics, postbiotics are safer because they reduce the chance of microbial translocation and infection and shield against any negative effects that probiotics can have in an environment where inflammation is already prevalent. Probiotic use has also been linked to the spread of antibiotic resistance genes and the inhibition of normal colonization by other microorganisms. The long-term effects of early colonization with dominant strains of probiotics on immune system development and microbiota maturation remain unknown.

3.15. Postbiotics

Though a precise understanding of the mechanisms of action remains unclear, data suggests that postbiotics have a variety of bioactive effects, such as immune function modification, anti-inflammatory response, and antibacterial activity. Postbiotics are made up of a variety of compounds that can be categorized into lipids, proteins, cofactors, organic acids, carbohydrates, vitamins, and complex molecules like lipoteichoic acids and muropeptides generated from peptidoglycan. Although some studies have looked into Streptococcus and Faecalibacterium species as a source of postbiotics, the majority of postbiotics are derived from Lactobacillus and Bifidobacterium strains (Vinderola, Sanders, and Salminen, 2022). The first cells in the gut lumen to come into contact with bacteria are intestinal epithelial cells. The mucus layer, the glycocalyx on the microvilli of absorptive intestinal epithelial cells, and the tight cell junctions act as physical barriers to prevent the infiltration of intestinal microbes. Specifically, mucins make up the majority of mucus. The inner layer serves as a wall to prevent bacterial adherence and invasion of the underlying epithelial cells. It is firmly adhered to the intestinal epithelium and is devoid of microorganisms. The outer layer contains many intestinal microbes and is created when the host or bacteria break down highly polymerized gel-like MUC2, the primary secretory mucin, through glycosidic and proteolytic processes. Postbiotics help restore intestinal homeostasis by generating bacteriocins, a diverse class of antimicrobial peptides with bacteriostatic or bactericidal properties. It has been shown that the medium composition influences the production of bacteriocin and that the right ratio of carbon and nitrogen sources can increase it. Bacteriocin influences the composition of the microbiota and the function of the immune system by preferentially competing with specific bacterial strains. It has been demonstrated that several additional postbiotic substances, including enzymes and organic acids, prevent the proliferation of infections. *Lactobacillus reuteri* produces reuterin, a potent antipathogenic molecule that has been shown to mediate the health advantages associated with this bacterium. It has been shown that reuterin suppresses the growth of bacteria, causing oxidative stress in cells and aiding in the regulation of a balanced gut microbiota. It has been demonstrated that bacterial exopolysaccharides mediate part of the advantageous effects linked to probiotics like bifidobacteria. Exopolysaccharides are repeated mono-or oligosaccharide subunits connected by various glycosidic bonds. Because of this, the structural variety of these molecules might affect their biological function. Since they operate as a fermentable substrate for other bacteria, exopolysaccharides associated with the cell surface of bifidobacteria appear to have an impact on the composition of the microbiota. It has been demonstrated that the bacterial exopolysaccharide produced by a strain of *Bifidobacterium breve* can lower the levels of colonization of the gut pathogen *Citrobacter rodentium*, most likely by facilitating the formation of biofilms (Fanning et al., 2012). The absence of surface exopolysaccharide expression has been linked to higher pathogen concentrations

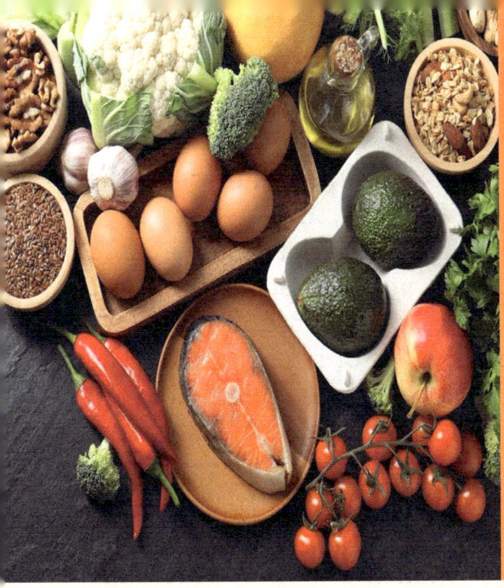

Chapter 4

BIOACTIVE FOODS AND CHRONIC GI DISEASES

Contents

4.1. Introduction

For the majority of patients, nutrition has a major impact on total metabolism due to its biochemical effects. It is evident that dietary choices influence the development of common pathophysiological problems like metabolic syndrome, and insulin resistance, and its consequences. These dynamics, however, can also be seen as a chance to reverse immunological reactivity using possible strategies that patients can adopt daily. Nutrient absorption, immunological protection against foreign agents, development, physiologic repair, neurohormone control, and stress management are all significantly influenced by the digestive tract. Anyplace in the gastrointestinal tract can have disorders that impact general health and body function (Oshima and Miwa, 2016). Low levels of buffering minerals like magnesium and potassium indicate that a diet that promotes metabolic acidosis might lead to toxin accumulation in the body. Many extensive studies with thousands of participants have documented the relationship between insulin resistance and metabolic acidosis, osteoporosis, coronary heart disease, and cardiometabolic risk, as well as cancer. The average American diet lacks the minerals and fiber needed to prevent or buffer the accumulation of metabolic acids and aid in the removal of harmful waste products. Consequently, as the intracellular environment grows increasingly acidic, mineral-depleted, and proton-rich, the alkaline cellular reserves decrease. Metabolic acidosis manifests as diabetes and metabolic syndrome, osteopenia, and osteoporosis, and depression. Because metabolic acidosis reduces the proton gradient, which is essential for cell energy, it is linked to a range of clinical disorders in the body. The ATP: ADP ratio aids as a measure of cell energy.

The common complaint from patients to their primary care physician is low energy. Even slight increases in acidity affect the body's capacity to produce energy and safely eliminate pollutants. Some researchers have connected metabolic acidosis to immune dysfunction syndrome and chronic fatigue. It has been shown that fibromyalgia and chronic pain that is not relieved by painkillers contain acidic end products that directly irritate and inflame nerve muscle end plates. Another important component of osteoporosis is an excess of acid in the cells. The impact of the acid-alkali balance on the integrity, health, and structure of the skeleton is among the best examples of metabolic sensitivity. Since skeletal muscles contain the majority of the accessible mineral reserves, they are extremely sensitive to even slight pH variations. Increased osteoclastic activity and decreased osteoblastic function are caused by even a 10% pH drop, which amplifies the loss of bone mineral. The single layer of epithelial cells that makes up the intestinal mucosa divides the body from the gut lumen, which contains commensal flora and potentially pathogenic antigens. Because of oral tolerance, normal intestinal mucosa is not hypersensitive to commensal flora. By generating the immunosuppressive cytokines interleukin (IL)-10, transforming growth factor (TGF)-β, and secretory IgA, gut-associated lymphoid tissue shields the intestinal mucosa from intestinal antigens. Chronic nonspecific inflammatory bowel disorders (IBDs) are ulcerative colitis (UC) and Crohn's disease (CD). The number of people afflicted with these diseases has been rising, with North America and Western Europe seeing the largest increases. While CD mostly affects the terminal ileum and/or the colon, UC primarily affects the colon and rectum. Although the precise pathophysiology of IBD is unknown, environmental variables, genes associated with disease susceptibility, and dysregulated immune response play a vital role in the disease development.

4.2. Pathology

Studies on CD in humans and mice have demonstrated that intestinal lamina propria cells express more T-helper 1 (Th1) cytokines (Parronchi et al., 1997). Th17 cells are involved in UC. Disturbed epithelial barrier function may elicit pathologic responses from the normal mucosal immune system, and deregulation of the mucosal immune system in these diseases results in excessive immunologic responses to the normal microflora or changes in the composition of intestinal microflora. To detect any indications of intestinal foreign agents, intestinal dendritic cells stretch their transepithelial dendrites into the intestinal lumen. The majority of tissue-resident mononuclear phagocytes, or macrophages, are involved in the polarization of innate and adaptive immunizations in addition to the identification and eradication of microorganisms. Intestinal macrophages secrete pro and anti-inflammatory cytokines, including TNF-α, IFN-γ, IL-6, and reactive oxygen species (ROS), as well as anti-inflammatory cytokines, i.e., IL-10 and TGF-β. While the human gut does not have many CD^{14+} cells, the intestinal mucosa of individuals with CD and UC has a substantial increase in these cells. In response to stimuli involving commensal bacteria, CD^{14+} and CD^{33+} cells released high levels of proinflammatory cytokines, including IL-12/IL-23p40, IL-23, TNF-α, and IL-6. These CD-derived macrophages are derived from bone marrow monocytes. IFN-γ in the CD mucosa caused abnormal macrophage differentiation, which in turn produced an excess of IL-23. In 60–70% of CD patients, a granuloma composed of lymphocytes and epithelioid macrophages was discovered in the digestive system (Amarnath et al., 2021). IBD was highly prevalent in the USA, Canada, and Western Europe at first, then as economies developed, it spread to East Europe and Eastern Asia. Westernized foods typically include dairy products, animal fats, meats, and other dietary components. The dietary characteristics that were linked to a higher chance of relapse for UC patients included a high meat or alcohol intake. One of the causes is that milk and animal products cause the large intestine to create hydrogen sulfide, a cell toxin that originates from bacteria and is detrimental to the colon.

4.3. Fish Oils

The long-chain n-3 polyunsaturated fatty acids eicosapentaenoic (EPA) and docosahexaenoic (DHA) are abundant in fish oils. α-linolenic acid, the precursor fatty acid, is abundant in the tissues of linseed and green plants. The majority of vegetable oils are high in linoleic acid that serves as an intermediate form of arachidonic acid. Prostaglandin E2, an eicosanoid produced from arachidonic acid, is proinflammatory. Fish oils (Figure 4.1) are therefore regarded as anti-inflammatory. Human macrophages secreted proinflammatory cytokines such as TNF-α, IL-8, and IL-1β in response to palmitic and stearic acids, but not to shorter-chain saturated fatty acids.

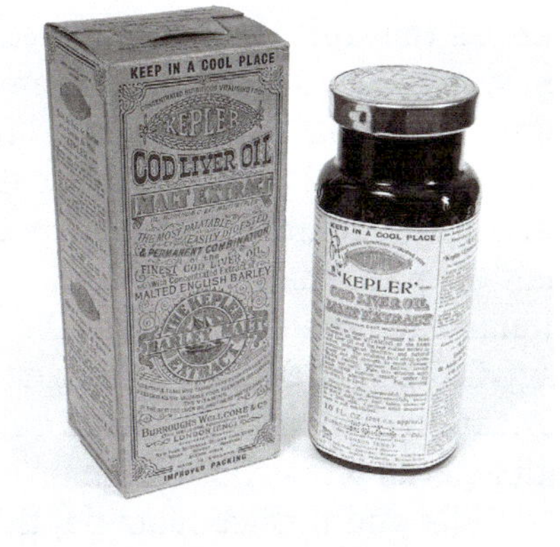

Figure 4.1. *Fish oils.*

Source: https://upload.wikimedia.org/wikipedia/commons/8/81/Kepler_Cod_Liver_Oil%2C_by_Burroughs_Wellcome_%26_Co_Wellcome_L0016947.jpg, Creative Commons License.

A dietary glutamine supplement prevented the generation of TNF-α and IL-8 in colitis caused by trinitrobenzene sulfonic acid. Rats with chemically induced experimental colitis were protected against by dietary glycine. Dietary histidine has been shown to have anti-inflammatory effects on macrophage and monocyte production of TNF-α, which may be one of the methods by which it suppresses an inflammatory response. Intestinal epithelial cell lines exposed to TNF-α or oxidative stress were unable to produce as much IL-8 in response to histidine's ability to scavenge hydroxyl radicals (OH). Therefore, diets containing amino acids may have an impact on how IBD develops. It is estimated that there are 500–2000 species in the human gut microflora, with a population of 10^{13}–10^{15} (Marć, Jastrząb and Mytych, 2022). Intestinal microbes play a role in the pathophysiology of inflammatory bowel disease (IBD).

4.4. Genetics of Irritable Bowel Syndrome

It is believed that IBD is a complicated genetic disease. Many CD susceptibility genes were discovered by genome-wide scans. Mutations in CARD15/NOD2 (nucleotide-binding oligomerization domain 2) were present in Caucasian CD patients. As a mediator between intracellular bacterial sensing and the onset of autophagy, CARD15/NOD2 or nucleotide-binding oligomerization domain 2 activity is believed to have antibacterial properties in human intestinal epithelial cells and intracellular peptidoglycan receptors. A possible susceptibility gene for CD is the single nucleotide polymorphism of NOD2, which triggers nuclear factor NF-kB. Intestinal epithelial cells express CARD15/NOD2, which stimulates the transcription of human beta-defensin (HBD)-2. The ileal Paneth cell defensins, HD-2 and HD-3, which are antimicrobial peptides, were reduced in CD patients with a NOD2 gene mutation. The intracellular catabolic process of autophagy eliminates a cell's own defective proteins and organelles through the lysosome. Pathological conditions like the granuloma formation that is commonly observed in CD can be caused by impaired autophagy. In CD, there are many single nucleotide polymorphisms in genes linked to autophagy. The elimination of bacterial invasion is significantly aided by the autophagy-related 16 like 1 or ATG16L1 protein that NOD2 recruits to the plasma membrane. It is believed that ATG16L1 and NOD2-regulated autophagy defects play an important role in the pathophysiology of CD.

4.5. Reactive Oxygen and Nitrogen Species

Many acute and chronic inflammatory diseases have been linked to reactive oxygen and nitrogen species pathogenesis. Some processes transform oxygen into reactive metabolites through reduction: the respiratory chain reaction, which produces toxic metabolites in the presence of oxygen, the activated phagocytic cells via nicotinamide adenine dinucleotide phosphate (NADPH) oxidase in the membranes of neutrophils and macrophages, and the ischemic-reperfusion processes, which result in the conversion of adenosine triphosphate to hypoxanthine and xanthine dehydrogenase by xanthine oxidase. Superoxide anion (O^{-}_{2}) is the first oxygen metabolite to be created when oxygen is reduced by one electron (Elstner, 1987). A series of reactions then produce hydrogen peroxide (H_2O_2), OH, hypochlorous acid (HOCl), and water (H_2O). H_2O_2 or superoxide generation may directly damage tissue. It is also believed that oxidants that are secondarily derived, like OH and HOCl, are the main mediators of tissue damage. Mucosal oxidases, such as xanthine, amine, and aldehyde oxidases, as well as NADPH oxidase, which is present in the phagocytic leukocytes (macrophages) of the mucosal lamina propria, are sources of reactive oxygen species (ROS) in the gastrointestinal tract. The OH produced by the iron-catalyzed reaction between superoxide and H_2O_2 appears to be the last mediator of toxicity.

ROS is essential to cell normal operation. The respiratory chain maintains the cell activity, while ROS are used by phagocytic cells to eliminate ingested bacteria. The metabolism of arachidonic acid, the cyclooxygenase and lipoxygenase systems, and the use of oxygen are critical for maintaining cellular homeostasis, protecting cell membranes, and triggering the immune system. Excessive ROS generation can occasionally damage cells. Oxygen radicals

O_2 and OH^- have the ability to cause tissue damage through lipid peroxidation, membrane instability, DNA damage, and the deactivation of proteolytic enzymes and protease inhibitors. Respiratory burst of peripheral blood monocytes and PMNL or polymorphonuclear leukocytes in UC were reported to be strongly correlated with disease progression. When comparing the chemiluminescence activity of CD patients to that of controls, a substantial increase was only observed in the monocyte fraction and not in the PMNL fraction. Patients with anal fistulas had significantly greater levels of monocyte chemiluminescence in CD. The chemiluminescence values of PMNL from CD patients with and without anal fistula, however, did not differ significantly. Both in UC and controls, priming neutrophils with lipopolysaccharide (LPS) or bacterial lipoprotein boosted superoxide generation in a dose-dependent manner. There were no variations in the amount of superoxide produced by the UC and the controls. Nonetheless, there was a correlation found between the Crohn's disease activity index (DAI) and C-reactive protein and the whole blood luminol-enhanced chemiluminescence. The addition of dimethylthiourea, azide, SOD, and deferoxamine caused the chemiluminescence levels to decrease. A peptide called interleukin-8 (IL-8) causes neutrophils to emit reactive oxygen species (ROS) in addition to causing them to chemotaxis. When colonic mucosa biopsy specimens from patients with active UC were compared to controls and patients with inactive UC, the levels of IL-8 and myeloperoxidase (MPO) in the tissue culture medium were considerably greater. When compared to controls and biopsy specimens in inactive UC, the ROS of the active UC specimens as determined by luminol-dependent chemiluminescence were significantly higher. MPO levels and luminol-dependent chemiluminescence were strongly linked with IL-8 levels (Freitas et al., 2010). In IBD patients, the percentage of activated platelets in the peripheral blood was higher. When there was no platelet–PMNL interaction, there was no discernible difference in the amounts of ROS produced by PMNL between UC patients and normal controls (NC). The activated platelets from UC patients increased the quantity of ROS generation. These findings showed that the development of intestinal lesions in CD may be influenced by the excessive active oxygen species generated by monocytes and macrophages. It has been demonstrated that intestinal macrophages from IBD patients respond more favorably to stimulation for the generation of O^-_2 than do peripheral blood monocytes. ROS generation was both activated and enhanced in intestinal macrophages from IBD patients. Through activation of the phagocyte-associated, ROS-producing NADPH oxidase, there will be an increase in the production of ROS within the tissue as a result of the inability to effectively regulate the activation of tissue macrophages as well as the recruitment and activation of phagocytic leukocytes such as neutrophils, eosinophils, and monocytes. Under normal circumstances, the majority of tissues have enough concentrations of non-enzymatic antioxidants like α-tocopherol, ascorbate, and sulfur as well as protective enzymatic molecules like SOD, catalase, and GSH peroxidase. Most of the harmful oxidants will be broken down by these compounds. However, UC had lower concentrations of these compounds. Overproduction of ROS has the potential to overcome defenses, causing oxidative damage to tissues and cells. The primary source of harmful ROS is thought to be phagocytic leukocytes.

The latent membrane-associated NADPH oxidase is activated by proinflammatory substances that interact with the phagocyte plasma membrane, including cytokines, leukotriene B4, platelet-activating factor, complement components, and bacterial products. When compared to healthy tissues, intestinal macrophages from CD patients had higher expression of the enzyme oxidase. Compared to neutrophils from healthy controls, people with UC may produce higher amounts of superoxide. Therefore, in UC patients, increased superoxide production can be attributed to both vascular endothelium permeability and monocyte invasion of the mucosa. PMNL and monocyte activation lead to increased production of HOCl, a powerful antioxidant, from MPO-catalyzed Cl oxidation by H_2O_2. Further, O_2 and H_2O_2 are less hazardous than HOCl, which has the oxidizing equivalents of H_2O_2. HOCl is a chlorinating and oxidizing chemical that reacts randomly with nucleotides, DNA, polyunsaturated fatty acids, sulfhydryls, and aromatic amino acids. ROS have the potential to indirectly induce epithelial and mucosal damage by modulating the equilibrium between the intestinal tissue protease and antiprotease.

Protease inhibitors are made inactive by neutrophil-derived oxidants like HOCl. The MPO-H_2O_2-chloride system is used by human neutrophils to produce chlorinated oxidants, which in turn activate collagenolytic metalloproteinase. The intestinal environment is made favorable for proteinase-mediated breakdown of the mucosal interstitial matrix and epithelial cells through the oxidative inactivation of protease inhibitors along with oxidant-mediated activation of metalloproteinase. A significant number of PMNL, monocytes, and lymphocytes are present in the inflammatory mucosa of colitis. The immune system's primary function is defense, and this defense involves activating Th1 cells and releasing proinflammatory cytokines from them as well as activating intestinal macrophages and other phagocytic leukocytes to release more proinflammatory cytokines. The body uses these cytokines as well as TNF-α, IL-1β, IL-22, and IL-23, among others, to defend itself against invasive microbes (Zhang et al., 2023). One important factor in the pathophysiology of IBD is believed to be the dysregulated immune system, which results in excessive production of proinflammatory cytokines and deficiency of inhibitory cytokines like TGF-β and IL-10.

4.6. The Biology of Inflammation

The intestine that is chronically inflamed experiences substantial oxidative damage. Since the administration of radical scavengers (oxypurinol), antioxidant enzymes like SOD, catalase, and enzyme inhibitors like sodium azide decreased ROS-related chemiluminescence, these increases in ROS were caused by neutrophil or monocyte-derived oxidants such as superoxide, H_2O_2, OH, and hypochlorite. Lipid hydroperoxide detoxification stops persistent intestinal inflammation. Depletion of endogenous oxidant defense components like ascorbate, β-carotene, β-tocopherol, and GSH as well as the regulatory, suppressive T lymphocytes are characteristics of individuals with UC. GSH is highly expressed in tissues. De novo production from precursor amino acids that contain sulfur, such as cysteine and methionine, and regeneration through the reduction of GSH disulfide, maintain normal amounts of GSH in cells. In inflammatory tissue, nitric oxide (NO) is known to have antagonistic effects. NO produced from inducible nitric oxide synthase or iNOS either directly or indirectly aids in the development and progression of tissue damage and inflammation. The oxidant ONOO is created when NO and O_2 interact. By directly inhibiting NADPH oxidase, NO can reduce the production of superoxide.

4.7. Models

The severe inflammation may be explained by the inhibition of NO generation and the resulting elevation of NADPH oxidase action. Using a tonometric balloon approach, rectal luminal NO levels were measured using the chemiluminescence technique. The results of some studies demonstrated that patients with active IBD had higher NO levels than healthy controls, who had lowered NO levels. Rectal NO levels in IBD patients who responded well to anti-inflammatory therapy were significantly lower and were linked with disease activity. In the rectal mucosa of IBD patients, there was a substantial increase in NO generation and iNOS expression compared to controls.

Some researchers used luminol-dependent chemiluminescence to detect MPO-mediated active oxidants and lucigenin-dependent chemiluminescence to detect superoxide anion to examine the effects of sulfasalazine and its metabolites, sulfapyridine, and 5-ASA and on respiratory burst of PMNL. At concentrations similar to clinical doses, they reduced PMNL-induced ROS. They can inhibit hypochlorous acid produced by neutrophils and scavenge a range of free radicals, demonstrating their strong antioxidant activity. The salicylates work as OH scavengers.

Curcumin, SOD, and fish oils are the three antioxidants that have been the subject of clinically successful trials for the treatment of UC in humans. To elucidate the functions of ROS in the pathophysiology of IBD, a range of experimental colitis models are used, including transgenic mice, acetic acid-induced colitis, trinitrobenzene sulfonic dextran sulfate sodium (DSS)-induced colitis and acid (TNBS)-induced colitis.

4.8. Experiments with Curcumin

Curcumin, a spice derived primarily from the rhizomes of the *Curcuma longa L* (Figure 4.2) plant that grows in South and Southeast Asia gives curries their distinct flavor. Anti-inflammatory, anti-angiogenic, antioxidant, anticarcinogenic, antibacterial, hepatoprotective properties are only a few of curcumin's advantageous properties (Xu et al., 2018). It has been demonstrated that the dietary derivative curcumin inhibits NF-kB activation. The heterodimer RelA (p65) and NF-kB1 (p50) subunits make up the NF-kB protype. The main NF-kB protein present in the nucleus of intestinal epithelial cells activated by cytokines is this heterodimer. IkB, the endogenous inhibitor of NF-kB, interacts with NF-kB in the cytoplasm to regulate NF-kB activation. Curcumin reduces the gene expression of intestinal epithelial cells following cytokine stimulation by blocking the signal that causes IKK activation without directly affecting NIK or IKK. IkBα phosphorylation and degradation, IKK activity, and NF-kB activation were inhibited when IKK activation was blocked. Curcumin also functions as a free radical scavenger and has anti-oxidative qualities. By adjusting NF-kB activation, ROS controls NF-kB activity in cells.

Rats were given 100 mg kg^{-1} of curcumin intraperitoneally for seven days in a row. This reduced the harmful effects of DSS and improved the inflammatory parameters. When compared to rats treated with DSS alone, pretreatment with curcumin before DSS administration produced a drop in the levels of serum TNF-α by approximately 46% and lowered the colonic MPO activity by approximately 57%. As compared to rats treated with DSS alone, the prior administration of curcumin before DSS boosted the colon GSH content by 117%, increased the colon GSH-S-transferase activity by roughly 79% and decreased the colon levels of malondialdehyde (MDA) by 56%. These findings imply that curcumin may protect against colitis by controlling the ratio of antioxidants to oxidants and modifying TNF-α release. Mice treated with curcumin before TNBS-induced colitis showed a considerable improvement in inflammation-induced colon mucosa MPO and MDA activities. The animals treated with curcumin showed a suppression of NF-kB activation in the colon mucosa. When TNBS-treated mice were given curcumin, their mucosal cell production of IL-12 mRNA was significantly suppressed, which decreased their capacity to produce IFN-γ. Curcumin may reduce NF-kB-mediated activation and binding to the p40-kB site as a means of inhibiting IL-12 production. By reducing inhibitory factor, I-kB kinase activity, curcumin has been demonstrated to prevent proinflammatory gene expression and cytokine-mediated NF-kB activation. These healing properties may be due to its capacity to eliminate reactive oxygen species (ROS) and nitrogen, which is demonstrated by decreased levels of superoxide anions, NO, MDA, and serine protease. Curcumin decreased the expression of iNOS and COX-2 and diminished the activation of p38 mitogen-activated protein kinases.

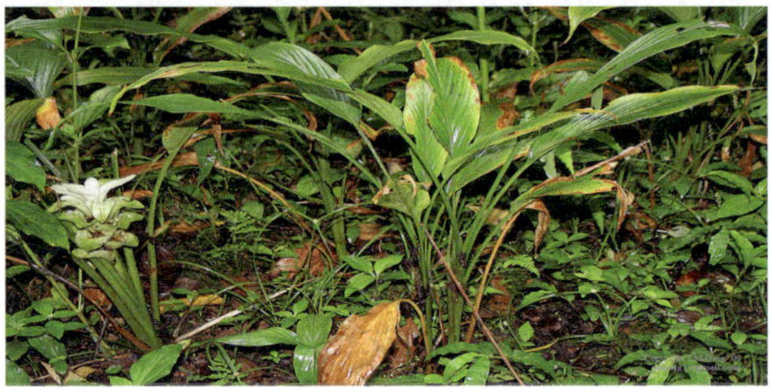

Figure 4.2. *Curcuma longa.*

Source: https://upload.wikimedia.org/wikipedia/commons/c/c9/Curcuma_longa_%28Haldi%29_Im_IMG_2441.jpg, Creative Commons License.

4.9. Research on Anti-oxidants

Among the proteins that are antioxidants is SOD. Superoxide dismutation to H_2O_2 is catalyzed by SOD and then detoxified by catalase or GSH peroxidase to produce oxygen and water (Vives-Bauza, et al., 2007). SOD is quickly eliminated from the kidney and does not bind to cellular membranes. Humans contain three different isoforms of SOD: extracellular (EC)-SOD, manganese (Mn)-SOD, and copper/zinc (Cu/Zn)-SOD. Cu/Zn-SOD has been studied as a potential treatment for IBD since it is a crucial antioxidant that is decreased in inflammatory colonic tissues. The experimental colitis was prevented from developing by the administration of Cu/Zn-SOD. These results suggested that SOD might have therapeutic value in the management of IBD. Cu/Zn-SOD has poor affinity in plasma and a short half-life of a few minutes, however, prevented any improvement in clinical trials conducted on patients with IBD in the early stages. Four phosphatidylcholine-derived molecules are covalently attached to each SOD dimmer in PC-SOD, a lecithinized human Cu/Zn-SOD. Some researchers attempted to elucidate the effects of PC-SOD and unmodified SOD on experimental colitis produced by 4% DSS. The PC-SOD-treated animals showed a considerable amelioration of colon shortening caused by inflammation and leukocyte infiltration. Higher PC-SOD dosages, however, had no appreciable impact on colon DAI. Superoxide anion levels generated by activated neutrophils were found to be lower in PC-SOD than in unmodified SOD. Only when catalase was also administered at the same time as PC-SOD did the elevated H_2O_2 levels in the DSS-treated mice decrease. The treatment of PC-SOD inhibited the elevated mRNA expression of TNF-α and IL-1β in DSS-induced colitis, but not that of IL-6 or IL-23p19. PC-SOD reduced intestinal ROS levels, which in turn inhibited TNF-αand IL-1β production and lessened the symptoms of colitis brought on by DSS. In DSS-induced colitis, treatment of both a low dose of PC-SOD and a high dose of PC-SOD with catalase reduced increased levels of NF-kB.

Transferring SOD genes is another way to elucidate the function of SOD. An isozyme of SOD called EC-SOD is mostly active in body fluids. Subcutaneous injections of syngeneic fibroblasts transduced retrovirally with the EC-SOD gene transfer were made into the mice with DSS-induced colitis. Treatment of colitis mice with SOD decreased enhanced expression of colonic lipid hydro peroxidation and MPO activity, as well as endothelium vascular cell adhesion molecule-1 and mucosal addressin cell adhesion molecule-1 in colitic interleukin-10 knockout mice. In the IL-10-deficient mice model, *Lactobacillus gasseri* expressing Mn-SOD was employed to treat colitis. When compared to untreated controls, *L. gasseri* generating Mn-SOD dramatically decreased inflammation in IL-10 defective mice. *L. gasseri* anti-inflammatory properties were linked to a decrease in neutrophil and macrophage infiltration (Oh et al., 2020). Rats with colitis brought on by TNBS were given a similar treatment utilizing *Lactococcus lactis and L. plantarum* that had been genetically modified to express SOD. Experimental colitis was treated with a variety of herbal treatments. The bark of the *Slippery elm* tree, sometimes known as redtree, is native to North America and is used to treat gastrointestinal tract irritation. An aromatic herb called fenugreek is claimed to help soothe irritable intestines. It has steroidal saponins, which are the building blocks for the body's synthesis of steroids. The tuberized root of the Mexican yam, a tropical perennial rich in starch and considered a staple meal in certain regions, has saponins in the form of Dioscorea. It is applied to the management of intestinal (gut) and joint inflammation. A flowering plant endemic to southern Africa is called *Devil's claw*. Ailments of the stomach and liver are treated with the tuberized secondary roots. It is claimed to have anti-inflammatory and analgesic qualities. It has flavonoids, which have been shown to scavenge free radicals.

4.10. Other Bioactives

Oxygen radicals can receive a hydrogen atom from plant phenols to create stable, inert chemicals. Tormentil grows throughout Europe. It is claimed to be useful in the management of intestinal irritation and diarrhea. It has a high tannin content, which is known for having strong superoxide-scavenging properties. Traditional Chinese medicine, known as *Wei tong ning*, is used to treat patients with peptic ulcers and other inflammatory intestinal conditions. Using luminol-enhanced chemiluminescence analysis, *in vitro* studies were conducted to evaluate the scavenging properties of these herbal medicines against oxygen radicals produced by mucosal biopsy specimens taken from individuals with active UC. All herbs, except for fenugreek, scavenged superoxide in a way similar to that of 5-ASA. Except for Mexican yam, all herbs showed a decrease in the amount of oxygen radicals generated from biopsy specimens.

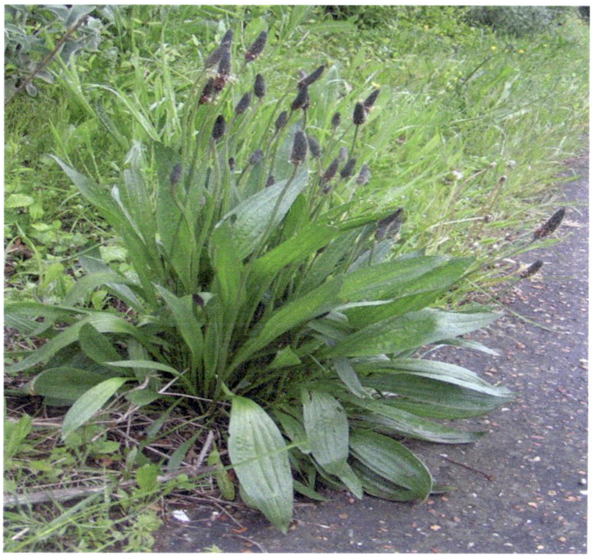

Figure 4.3. *Plantago lanceolata.*

Source: https://en.wikipedia.org/wiki/Plantago_lanceolata#/media/File:Ribwort_600.jpg, Creative Commons License.

Plantago lanceolata L. (Figure 4.3) is the source of acteoside, an herbal phenylethanoid that has been derived from plantain herb. Acteoside has anti-oxidative potential and suppresses 5-hydroxy-6, 8,11,14-eicosatetraenoic acid, leukotriene B, and other inflammatory chemicals. It suppresses 5-lipoxygenase and iNOS enzymatic activity that are present in neutrophils and macrophages. Acteoside considerably reduced colitis in cases with DSS-induced colitis. Acteoside treatment resulted in a prominent decrease in IFN-γ release from activated lymphocytes from colitis mice mesenteric lymph nodes. In colitis caused by DSS, mucosal tissue damage was reduced when acteoside was used to inhibit oxidative burst activity. Green tea has polyphenols and is a known antioxidant. Tempol is a metal-independent SOD mimetic and a membrane-permeable radical scavenger. Tempol significantly diminished the onset of diarrhea and body weight loss in rats with colitis produced by dinitrobenzene sulfonic acid (DNBS). This was linked to a decrease in the inflammatory colon level of lipid peroxidation and neutrophil infiltration. In mice with colitis caused by DSS, the colon shortening and damage score were temporarily mitigated.

In mice with colitis produced by DSS, edaravone, a free radical scavenger, decreased elevated levels of colonic MPO and serum IL-6. IAC is a novel low-molecular-weight radical scavenger that is reactive with the majority of radicals that are centered on carbon, nitrogen, and oxygen. In DNBS-induced colitis, IAC blocked the reduction of body weight growth, colonic damage and inflammation, and TNF-α levels (Vasina et al., 2009). Antioxidant regulator Prohibitin was found to be downregulated in colitis and overexpressed in intestinal epithelial cells that were cultivated. Oxidative stress was prevented for Prohibitin. In intestinal epithelial cells under oxidative conditions, it controls the expression of nuclear factor erythroid 2-related factor 2, a transcriptional regulator of oxidant responses. Prohibitin reduced damage and oxidative stress associated with inflammation through the initiation of nuclear factor erythroid 2-related factor 2. Allopurinol is a scavenger of free radicals produced by oxygen and is used to treat gout. Superoxide anions can be produced by xanthine oxidase by the conversion of hypoxanthine to xanthine and uric acid. Sulfasalazine, a superoxide anion scavenger, and methoxypolyethylene glycol: SOD greatly reduced the severity of inflammation in experimental colitis caused by the intracolonic injection of 5% acetic acid. Tungsten and pterin aldehyde, two xanthine oxidase inhibitors, did not reduce inflammation; however, allopurinol, another xanthine oxidase inhibitor, did reduce inflammation. The xanthine oxidase pathway is not a generator of ROS in this colitis model. The prevalent cellular antioxidant produced by animal cells, glutathione (GSH) is vital to cell biology and regulates how cells react to redox shifts brought on by reactive oxygen species (ROS). In the trans-sulfuration pathway, S-adenosylmethionine, a GSH precursor, is a necessary step between methionine and cysteine.

Mice treated with DSS showed improved colon lesions and higher body weights. When antioxidant-treated mice have blood levels of reduced GSH, elevated amyloid A, and TNF-α returns to normal. As a GSH precursor, N-acetylcysteine (NAC) decreased elevated levels of colonic MPO activity, ROS, TNF-α, and interleukin-1β. It raised GSH levels and PON1 activity. Though its low doses had no protective effects, some studies found that NAC significantly decreased the degree of colonic injury, most likely by controlling the formation of free radicals and suppressing inflammation. In rats treated with TNBS, NAC alone or in conjunction with 5-ASA reduced prostaglandin E2 levels and COX2 gene expression to control levels. In acetic acid-induced colitis, L-carnitine supplementation reduced MDA and MPO levels and enhanced histologic scores. L-carnitine supplementation raised SOD levels and stopped the depletion of lowered GSH levels without affecting catalase activity. iNOS is an enzyme that metabolizes reactive oxygen species and nitrogen. While N omega-nitro-L-arginine methyl ester (NAME), a nonselective NOS inhibitor, decreases oxidant levels, arginine raises NO levels. In TNBS-induced experimental colitis, the arginine-administered group had significantly higher levels of NO and thiobarbituric acid reactive substances (TBARS) than glycine-administered groups. These levels were reduced when NAME was administered to both glycine and L-arginine-administered groups. When arginine was given to the group instead of glycine, there was a considerable increase in both GSH levels and GSH peroxidase activity. Compared to arginine alone, the L-arginine + L-NAME group exhibited significantly increased Cu/Zn SOD activity (Ortiz et al., 2013). The severity of DSS-induced colitis was reduced in mice with iNOS genetic deficiency or in mice treated with a specific iNOS inhibitor. It was shown that intestinal inflammation is caused by different forms of superoxide produced by membrane-associated NADPH oxidase in active neutrophils and iNOS-derived NO. In experimental colitis, oxidant damage may be influenced by NO. However, the administration of L-NAME or aminoguanidine greatly lowered the healing of DSS-induced colonic lesions, and the co-administration of L-arginine significantly counteracted the effects of L-NAME. The NO generated by iNOS aided in the colonic lesions caused by DSS to heal.

4.11. IBD Management

The fish oil has both EPA and DHA. Many studies have examined the impact of omega-3 fatty acid-containing fish oil on the management of inflammatory bowel disease. Leukotriene B4 levels of rectal dialysates and prednisolone concentration decreased after four months of this supplement on therapy with prednisolone or sulfasalazine in UC patients. Some researchers conducted a trial involving 10 patients with mild to moderate UC. Four out of five patients on prednisolone were able to lower their steroid dose, and seven out of 10 patients showed moderate to remarkable improvement. Three patients, however, showed little to no improvement. The purpose of the other trial was to determine whether UC patients would benefit from combination therapy consisting of sulfasalazine and omega-3 fatty acid from fish oil. This investigation revealed no statistically significant alterations in any laboratory indicator, sigmoidoscopy, or histology scores. Researchers found that there was a decrease in oxidative stress in both the microsomal lipid peroxidation inhibition assay and total plasma antioxidant capacity. Many vegetable oils, such as those derived from corn, sunflower, and soybeans, as well as goods (products) manufactured from them, like margarines, contain substantial amounts of linoleic acid. Green plant tissues, several common vegetable oils, certain nuts, flaxseed, and flaxseed oil are all good sources of α-linolenic acid. Linoleic and α-linolenic acids together account for more than 95% of the PUFAs consumed in typical Western diets. However, linoleic acid intake is higher than that of α-linolenic acid.

Eicosanoids are derived from 20-carbon polyunsaturated fatty acids and are important mediators and regulators of inflammation and immunity (Calder, 2001). The arachidonic acid metabolism produces eicosanoids, which include prostaglandins (PGs), thromboxanes, leukotrienes, and other oxidized derivatives. Eicosanoids have sources that are specific to cells and stimuli, and they often have opposite (antagonistic) effects. They are involved in regulating the duration and strength of immunological and inflammatory responses. Therefore, the cells present, the type of stimulus, the time of eicosanoid production, the quantities of various eicosanoids generated, and the sensitivity of target cells and tissues to the eicosanoids formed will all influence the overall physiological or pathological outcome. Since ARA is present in immune cell membrane phospholipids in very high concentrations, it usually serves as the main precursor for eicosanoid mediators, which are created in higher quantities in response to cellular activation. As a result, the majority of the eicosanoids produced are those synthesized from arachidonic acid, such as PGE_2 and LTB_4. However, the specific eicosanoid profile varies depending on the type of cell involved and the type of stimulus; additionally, the profile will change over time as the stimulus changes. When laboratory mice are subjected to colitis induction, the intestinal mucosa produces inflammatory eicosanoids like

PGE_2 and LTB_4. Inflammatory eicosanoids, such as LTB_4, are found in higher concentrations in the intestinal mucosa of people with IBD. Due to its unique proinflammatory properties, which include triggering leukocyte infiltration and the subsequent release of inflammatory mediators, LTB_4 is most likely contributing to the pathophysiology of IBDs. This is corroborated by the protective activity of the LT biosynthesis inhibitor MK-886 against mucosal damage in rat colitis caused by acetic acid. There was a correlation between this impact and lower intestinal LTB_4 levels. Though there is evidence that PGE_2 may be protective, its involvement in IBD is less clear. For instance, in rat colitis brought on by acetic acid, indomethacin, an inhibitor of PG production, exacerbated mucosal damage. Moreover, the LT synthesis inhibitor raised PGE_2 concentrations in addition to decreasing LTB_4 concentrations in the colon, indicating that a change in ARA metabolism in favor of PGs is advantageous.

The mechanisms by which PGE_2 may have anti-inflammatory effects have been clearly demonstrated by recent studies. PGE_2 has been shown to induce 15-lipoxygenase, which promotes the formation of lipoxins, which have been found to have anti-inflammatory effects, and to inhibit 5-lipoxygenase, which reduces the production of the inflammatory 4-series LTs. Lipoxin A_4 homolog given orally reduced mortality and weight loss in mice given oral dextran sodium sulfate (DSS) to cause colitis at the same time. PGE_2 production is increased by ARA feeding and decreased by EPA or DHA feeding. Increased intake of EPA and DHA reduces the ARA content of immune cell phospholipids. These observations are consistent with the direct relationship between the ARA of phospholipids (immune cells) and the capacity of those cells to produce PGE_2. 12 weeks following oral administration of 1.5 g ARA per day, blood mononuclear cells in human volunteers produced more PGE_2 and LTB_4. Fish oil supplementation for a period of weeks to months has been shown to significantly reduce *ex vivo* PGE_2 and 4-series-LT production by human immune cells. The cyclooxygenase and lipoxygenase enzymes that generate eicosanoids also use EPA as a substrate. However, the mediators that are generated differ structurally from mediators formed from arachidonic acid, which affects their efficacy. Neutrophils from humans supplied with oral fish oil for several weeks and macrophages from mice fed fish oil have been used to demonstrate increased production of 5-series LTs. After DSS induction of colonic inflammation, transgenic mice with the *C. elegans* n-3 desaturase gene were able to convert n-6 to n-3 PUFAs, leading to an elevated n-3 PUFA content in their tissues. These mice were also shown to produce large amounts of PGE_3 within colonic tissue. Since mediators obtained from EPA are less biologically active than those derived from arachidonic acid, the generation of eicosanoids from EPA has functional relevance. Resolvins are also produced by EPA and DHA via routes involving the enzymes lipoxygenase and cyclooxygenase (Seki et al., 2009).

4.12. Mechanisms of Nutrition

Studies on animal nutrition and cell culture have shown that these mediators are immunomodulatory, inflammatory-resolving, and anti-inflammatory. Resolvin E1, for instance, which is derived from EPA, has been demonstrated to protect mice against chemically induced colitis. This protective effect has been linked to a decrease in granulocyte infiltration into colonic tissue as well as a reduction in the expression of several inflammatory genes, including TNF-α, IL-12p40, cyclooxygenase-2, and inducible nitric oxide synthase, in that tissue. Resolvin synthesis has been demonstrated to occur in *fat-1* mice in which colitis had been induced and is enhanced in laboratory rodents fed diets rich in fish oil.

Marine n-3 PUFAs have been demonstrated to have effects on inflammation that are not only mediated by modifications in the pattern of eicosanoids and other lipid mediators generated, but also by altering the production of inflammatory cytokines. It is possible that this effect is mediated by activation of important transcription factors that control the expression of genes linked to inflammation. Two transcription factors, peroxisome proliferator activated receptor or PPAR-γ and NFkB, are probably involved in inflammation. The primary transcription factor responsible for the upregulation of adhesion molecules, cyclooxygenase-2, and inflammatory cytokine genes is NFkB. When extracellular inflammatory stimuli are present, an inhibitory subunit of NFkB is phosphorylated, initiating a signaling cascade that activates NFkB and permits the translocation of the remaining NFkB dimer to the nucleus. Inflammatory gene expression is hence increased. According to several studies, NFkB is a known target for regulating intestinal inflammation. The second transcription factor, PPAR-γ, is thought to have anti-inflammatory properties and is likewise expressed in intestinal tissue. Reduced PPAR-γ expression is seen in colon biopsies of UC patients; increased sensitivity to chemically induced colitis is seen in PPAR-γ knockdown mice; and in mouse models, colitis is lessened by PPAR-γ agonists. Accordingly, it has been established that PPAR-γ overexpression is a target for reducing intestinal inflammation. An interesting interaction between these transcription factors results from the reaction that PPAR-γ not only directly controls the expression of inflammatory genes but also prevents NFkB from being activated.

4.13. Results From Cell Culture Research

Cultured human endothelial cells were shown to produce less IL-6 and IL-8 in response to endotoxins, and cultured monocytes were shown to produce less TNF-α in response to endotoxins. EPA or fish oil reduced the activation of NFkB induced by endotoxins in human monocytes (Allam-Ndoul et al., 2017). This was linked to a decrease in IkB phosphorylation, possibly as a result of a decrease in the activation of mitogen-activated protein kinases. These findings point to the direct effects of marine n-3 PUFAs on the expression of genes associated with inflammation via blocking the activation of the transcription factor NFkB. Research on fish oil-fed animals validates findings from cell culture about the impact of marine n-3 PUFAs on NFkB activation and the production of inflammatory cytokines. For instance, in murine spleen cells stimulated by endotoxins, giving fish oil reduced NFkB activation in comparison to feeding maize oil. Mice fed fish oil had lower levels of circulating TNF-α, IL-1β, and IL-6 in mice given endotoxin injections and lessened *ex vivo* production of TNF-α, IL-1β, and IL-6 by endotoxin-stimulated macrophages. Endotoxin-stimulated monocytes or mononuclear cells have been shown to produce less TNF-α, IL-1β, and IL-6 in many studies in healthy human volunteers when the diet is supplemented with fish oil, though not all studies support this finding.

Many fatty acids, including n-3 PUFAs, have been demonstrated in cell culture studies to have effects on T-cell functional responses and signaling. These effects have also been demonstrated to be dose-dependent and to be related to variations in the fatty acid (FA) composition of lymphocyte phospholipids. *In vitro* T-cell proliferation and IL-2 production have both been demonstrated to be inhibited by EPA and DHA. Reduced T-cell proliferative responses have also been documented in animal feeding trials employing relatively high doses of fish oil, EPA, or DHA. The physical state of the plasma membrane; variations in the profile of eicosanoid mediators, which affect T-cell function; and direct effects on transcription factor activation are some of the mechanisms thought to be involved. Since lipid rafts appear to be closely involved in T-lymphocyte responses to activation, there has been some recent focus on whether marine n-3 PUFAs influence T-cell functions via effects on lipid rafts. When mice were fed a diet high in omega-3 PUFA (polyunsaturated fatty acids), EPA, and DHA were incorporated into the lipids of the splenic T cell rafts, which was linked to a decrease in the amount of sphingomyelin. Therefore, one possible mechanism for protein displacement from rafts is the incorporation of n-3 PUFAs into membrane lipids. The step that is inhibited by marine n-3 PUFA treatment of T cells is phosphorylation of the signaling protein linker of activated T cells (LAT). At least *in vitro*, LAT displacement from rafts appears to be a molecular mechanism mediating the inhibition of T-cell responses by n-3 PUFAs. Research on animals has demonstrated that dietary fish oil influences early T-cell signaling events, such as the phosphorylation of phospholipase C-γ1, and it has connected functional changes like lowered proliferation and IL-2 production with modifications to T-cell rafts caused by dietary n-3 PUFAs. Patients with IBD who take fish oil supplements to their diets have an integration of long-chain n-3 PUFAs into their gut mucosal tissue. Many studies have shown that fish oil has anti-inflammatory effects on patients with IBD. These include decreased production of LTB_4 by neutrophils, decreased production of PGE_2 and thromboxane B_2 by colonic mucosa, and decreased production of PGE_2 and IFN-γ by blood mononuclear cells (Sheppe and Edelmann, 2021). Fish oil supplementation has been shown to have therapeutic benefits in UC in a few pilot studies.

4.14. Other Food Materials and IBD

Soy sauce is known as shoyu in Japanese. Japan creates a wide range of shoyu. The varying kinds and ratios of raw materials utilized, the kinds of microorganisms used, and the fermentation conditions all affect their features. Naturally brewed shoyu is made in Japan. Wheat is roasted and ground and moistened soybeans are boiled at high pressure and temperature. These two substances are combined with a tiny quantity of *Aspergillus oryzae* (Figure 4.4) or A. sojae seed mold.

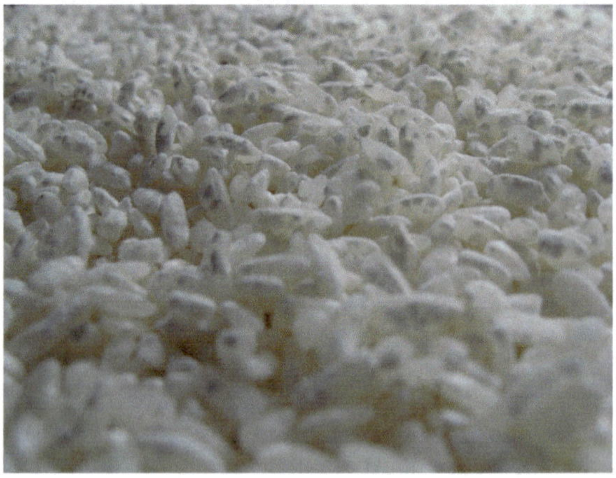

Figure 4.4. *Aspergillus oryzae.*

Source: https://upload.wikimedia.org/wikipedia/commons/c/c9/Aspergillus_oryzae_%28%E9%BA%B9%29.jpg, Creative Commons License.

This mixture is spread out on a large porous plate, and air is circulated through it at a predetermined temperature and moisture content to generate the ideal environment for the growth of mold and the synthesis of enzymes. The material grown in mold is called koji, and it is combined with a large amount of NaCl in water to create a mash known as moromi. The moromi, which has a 15% NaCl content, is kept for several months at ambient temperature or at a higher temperature in large tanks. After being fermented by yeasts and lactobacilli, the moromi is carefully matured. To make soy sauce (shoyu), the aged moromi is pressed and the liquid portion (raw soy sauce) is pasteurized. Since microbial proteolytic enzymes totally break down the proteins of the raw materials into peptides and amino acids during fermentation, soy sauce is free of allergens. On the other hand, soybean cell wall-derived polysaccharides are resistant to enzymatic hydrolysis and persist even after fermentation. To better understand the properties of the polysaccharides in soy sauce, researchers thoroughly examined and purified the polysaccharides. One of the primary basic components for soy sauce, the cell wall polysaccharides of soybeans, have a high galacturonic acid content and are only weakly degraded by mold enzymes in the koji and moromi stages.

These polysaccharides are known as shoyu polysaccharides (SPS) and account for about 1% of the soy sauce. Even while polysaccharides like pectic compounds have been known to be present in soy sauce for more than 30 years, research into their biological activity is still lacking. In placebo-controlled clinical trials, scientists recently showed that SPS has strong antiallergic effects both *in vitro* and *in vivo*, and oral supplementation of SPS was a useful intervention for patients with allergic rhinitis. It was discovered that SPS regulates the intestinal immune system as well as the balance of Th1/Th2 cell responses. SPS was discovered to improve iron absorption and lower increased levels of triacylglycerol in both animal and human trials when its nutritional roles in the gastrointestinal tract were further investigated. About 3–5 billion people are affected by iron deficiency, primarily women of reproductive age, newborns, and small children. It is a serious health issue in underdeveloped countries. The serious type of iron deficiency is anemia. Reduced intestine solubility and the presence of inhibitors like phytic acid from diets high in cereals may be the cause of reduced iron bioavailability. Food fortification is frequently thought to be the most economical long-term strategy for lowering the incidence of iron deficiency. Soy sauce is a popular traditional condiment in China, Thailand, and Vietnam, which makes it a potential option for usage as an iron transporter. Due to its high consumption and low cost, soy sauce is the recommended food condiment for iron fortification with rice meals in Southeast Asia, where iron (Fe) deficiency is a serious public health issue. In clinical trials, some researchers documented the beneficial effects of soy sauce on iron absorption. NaFeEDTA has a better rate of absorption in the human body, fewer side effects, and less of an impact on the bioavailability of other minerals when compared to regularly used Fe salt fortificants. Since then, China, Thailand, and Vietnam have reported success rates with the use of NaFeEDTA-fortified soy sauce and fish sauce in anemic women and children (Laillou et al., 2016). It is interesting to note that, regardless of its mode of action, soy sauce added to a rice dish seems to improve iron absorption. The mechanism this influence on iron absorption is yet unknown, although these findings may be somewhat relevant to iron nutrition in Asian countries where rice is a major staple food. It has been noted that soybeans have a negative impact on the absorption of iron from a mixed diet and have a low bioavailability of iron when consumed alone. High molecular weight protein would prevent the bioavailability of iron; however, the exact mechanism of action is unknown, probably through the creation of comparatively stable protein–iron aggregates. Because amino acids and short peptides are broken down by microbial hydrolyses during long-term fermentation, soy sauce is devoid of high-molecular-weight proteins. Since fermented soy sauce lacks the iron bioavailability inhibitors found in other soybean products, researchers showed that soy sauce had an important effect on the absorption of iron (Fe) from a rice meal. Likewise, miso, a fermented soybean product, enhanced iron bioavailability. Therefore, in societies where rice is the main food, historically fermented soybean products like miso and shoyu (soy sauce) would add to iron nutrition. Fermented soy sauce ingredients may play a role in the stimulating effect on iron absorption, even though the exact mechanism is still unknown. To further understand the stimulating properties of SPS as a useful dietary ingredient derived from soy sauce, some researchers investigated its ability to bind iron as well as its impact on animal and human iron absorption. Iron deficiency is frequently caused by low iron bioavailability from diets that appear to contain adequate levels rather than by insufficient intake. Nonheme iron is the main source of iron in these diets; its bioavailability is dependent on the type of iron consumed and how soluble it is in the digestive system. Dietary ligands that produce low solubility chelates are thought to decrease iron bioavailability, whereas those that form soluble iron chelates at intestinal pH values are thought to promote bioavailability. Many research studies have examined the impact of dietary fiber on iron bioavailability. Diets high in fiber have been found to reduce iron absorption in certain trials, but not in others. Pectin is a significant dietary polysaccharide that dissolves in water and has carboxylic groups that can bind to mineral ions to form complexes. Pectin in diets may decrease the bioavailability of minerals because the free carboxyl groups in the galacturonic acid units can form complexes with polyvalent cations such as Ca, Mg, Zn, and Fe. Nevertheless, research conducted *in vivo* revealed that pectin enhanced the absorption of iron, indicating that variations in the molecular weight and level of esterification of pectins impact their solubility and strength of mineral binding.

4.15. Final Points on Soy Sauce

Inorganic iron, in contrast to heme iron, must be dissolved in the digestive system to be properly absorbed. Soy sauce-derived SPS improved intestinal iron absorption by making inorganic iron more soluble (Qiao et al., 2022). In the stomach, for instance, ferrous, and ferric ions dissolve at low pH levels, whereas in the intestinal tract, they precipitate at neutral pH levels. Ferrous and ferric ions dissolve at neutral pH in the presence of SPS. SPS would create the combination Fe-SPS, which would increase iron solubility at neutral pH. In the small intestine, for example, at a neutral pH, soy sauce SPS would act as an iron stabilizer. SPS reduced iron excretion into the feces of rats fed anemic diets lacking in iron for two weeks, hence improving iron absorption and pooling in organs including the liver and spleen. After four weeks of treatment, serum iron, hematocrit, and hemoglobin levels were considerably higher in the SPS-administered group compared to the placebo-administered group in a double-blind, placebo-controlled clinical research of healthy women. Following a 4-week course of treatment, standard blood tests, which measure hepatic and renal function as well as protein and lipid concentrations, did not reveal any major abnormalities. Soy sauce can be used as an anti-anemic in daily life, and its SPS is safe and should encourage the fortification of meals with iron. The prevalence of lifestyle-related diseases like diabetes, hyperlipidemia, and hypertension has been rising rapidly in rich nations. Obesity is one of the major risk factors for a number of ailments. The main cause of obesity is dietary excess in lipids. Reducing lipid intake is a sensible nutritional measure given the link between dietary lipids and obesity and even heart disease. Nutritional therapy is crucial and may be the first line of treatment. Blocking the intestinal ability to absorb fat or raising the metabolic rate and fat oxidation are efficient strategies to avoid obesity.

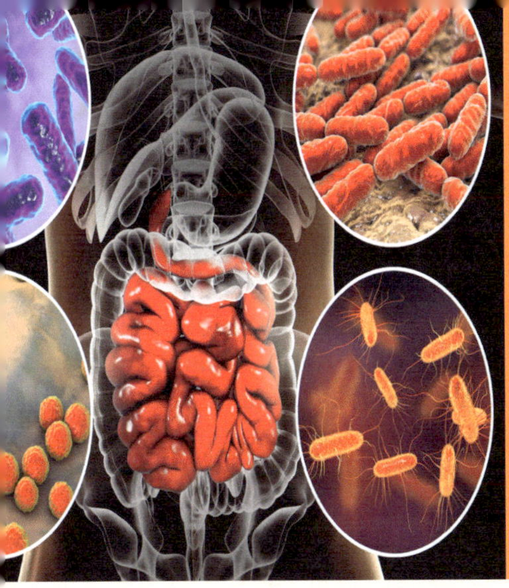

Chapter 5

GI DISEASES AND DIETARY INTERVENTIONS

Contents

5.1. Introduction

The gastrointestinal tract is a system that exists between the body's internal and external environments. The mouth, which has similar physical characteristics with the skin is where the GI tract begins. The mucosa is made up of a single layer of cells and becomes less complex as it develops. The tight junction proteins firmly bind a single layer of cells together in the intestine. Because the vast intestinal surface is covered in both gut-associated lymphoid tissue (GALT) (Figure 5.1) and mucosa-associated lymphoid tissue (MALT), it is now recognized as an important immune organ.

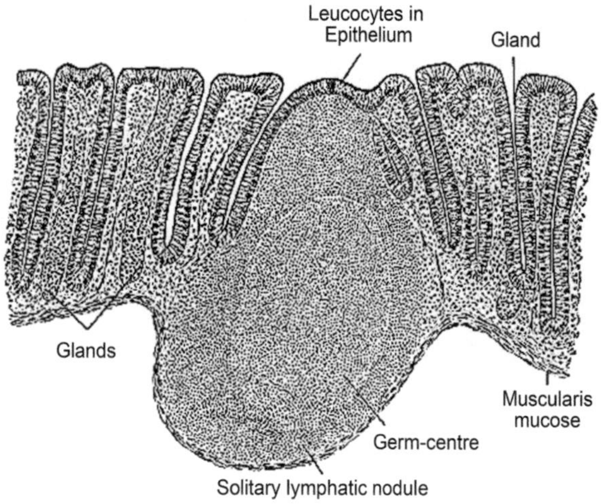

Figure 5.1. Gut-associated lymphoid tissue.

Source: https://upload.wikimedia.org/wikipedia/commons/5/5c/Gray1082.png, Creative Commons License.

The GI tract contains an important barrier system for its own protection: the glycocalyx and mucus layer (Corfield, 2015). This system is necessary because of the presence of enzymes for digestion and external pollutants. Both offer defense against pathogen invasion and detrimental damage. In order to prevent direct contact between the mucosa and the many microorganisms that cohabit along the GI tract, mucus must be present. The microbiota of the human gastrointestinal system is thought to consist of 10^{14} different bacterial species. The various microbial communities found in the GI tract, such as fungi, viruses, parasites, and primarily bacteria, make up the microbiota. The mucins, a family of glycoproteins made by goblet cells, generate the intestinal mucus and provide a home for commensal bacteria. Bacteria in the GI tract can either live freely or attach themselves to mucus to create biofilms, which are intricate microbial communities adhered to surfaces. Prebiotics, such as inulin-type fructans, influence the microbiota. Prebiotic use has been shown to decrease pathogen *Salmonella enterica* subsp. enterica serovar Typhimurium and increase mucosa-associated bifidobacteria, which may promote health, in rats implanted with human fecal microbiota. The administration of prebiotics also caused modifications to the mucosal architecture, such as a thicker mucus layer, an increase in villus height, and a decrease in crypt depth.

Drug-associated mucositis is an inflammation that can disrupt the GI system as a whole, significantly affecting quality of life and having clinical implications. Mucositis is an adverse event that frequently occurs in cancer patients receiving radiation therapy and/or chemotherapy. Many factors, such as chemotherapy plus radiation, aggressive chemotherapy in hematopoietic stem cell transplantation (HSCT) patients, patients whose primary tumor originated in the oral cavity, oropharynx, nasopharynx, or salivary glands, influence the incidence of mucositis. Oral and GI mucositis, which mostly affects the small intestine, are the two main types of mucositis. Fluorouracil, methotrexate, cisplatin, and irinotecan are the drugs that cause mucositis frequently. Diarrhea, nausea, vomiting, abdominal pain, malabsorption, and ensuing loss of body weight are the primary symptoms. Because of secondary infections and symptom management, mucositis is linked to higher hospital expenses. There is no effective treatment or prevention regimen for mucositis, despite its clinical significance. Innovative approaches, such as incorporating chemotherapy drugs into liposomes that are pH-sensitive appear to be better in mitigating the adverse effects of chemotherapy. Erythematous mucosal lesions are a characteristic of mild mucositis inflammation. On the other hand, ulcerative lesions that pierce the submucosal layer and cause excruciating pain and sharp inflammatory responses are also linked to the condition when the inflammation is severe.

These symptoms intensify and lead to increased mucosal cell death, which compromises mucosal integrity and causes lesions that eventually become ulcerations, which are more vulnerable to bacterial colonization and, as a result, more immunological activation. Severe pain follows these symptoms, and the entry of microbes that are already in the GI tract can cause sepsis and bacteremia in extreme cases. Mucositis is caused by an inflammatory reaction. The final biological stage of the disease is composed of the stimulus for healing that begins when cancer therapy is stopped. There is conflicting evidence on the role of GI microbiota in the onset or severity of mucositis. However, it has been shown in clinical research that the microbiota composition alters as a result of cancer therapy, with a drop in the overall quantity and diversity of bacteria, including a decline in Lactobacillus and Bifidobacteria, and an increase in pathobionts. Rats with mucositis also displayed altered microbiota, including elevated levels of *E. coli*. In comparison to ordinary mice, GF mice that were given irinotecan to produce mucositis displayed reduced inflammatory responses (Ribeiro et al., 2016).

5.2. Mucositis

Research on using prebiotics and dietary fiber as a different approach to treat or possibly lessen mucositis began a few years ago. Pectin-supplemented enteral diets produced interesting outcomes in rats with methotrexate-induced mucositis. Pectin-treated animals exhibited decreased intestinal MPO levels, decreased body weight loss, and decreased permeability in the colon and distal small bowel. An improved microbiome profile and decreased plasma endotoxin levels were observed. GBF (Germinated barley foodstuff) was also effective in reducing the chemotherapeutic agent-induced diarrhea, mucosal injury, bacterial translocation, and increase in MPO activity in the animal models. Sodium alginate is a different type of fiber that is not commonly found in human diets. It is a water-soluble dietary fiber that is produced from seaweed and is used to stop the reduction of RBC or red blood cell, hemoglobin, and hematocrit levels in mucositis rats. This may have other benefits that need to be investigated further. Mucositis is linked to radiation therapy as well as chemotherapy. Rats exposed to radiation experienced severe weight loss, diarrhea, and histological damage similar to humans. In radiation-induced mucositis rats, the histological profile was improved by the use of synbiotics containing *Lactobacillus acidophilus*, *Lactobacillus delbrueckii subsp. bulgaricus*, *Lactobacillus sporogenes*, and *Saccharomyces cerevisiae* in addition to glucooligosaccharides and a complex of vitamin B. The application of synbiotic treatment or FOS (fructooligosaccharides) alone worsened the clinical symptoms of the condition while lowering MPO levels in jejunum samples. There is not much information on using fiber to cure mucositis in humans. Promising results were shown in a trial that included enteral supplementation of glutamine, fiber, and oligosaccharide (GFO). The application of some molecules in mucositis has also been studied since the impact of dietary fiber and prebiotics is dependent on the generation of SCFAs (short-chain fatty acids) and the modification of the microbiota. SCFAs decreased intestinal irritation and minimized intestinal damage in mice in the 5-FU experiments (Ferreira et al., 2012). SCFAs might be a useful adjuvant for conditions affecting the colon and small intestine that needs further research.

5.3. Zataria multiflora Boiss (ZM)

Zataria multiflora Boiss (ZM) is a thyme-like plant in the Lamiaceae family. Several scientists have assessed its chemical composition. The dried aerial parts of ZM, particularly the leaves, are frequently used as a favorite condiment in Persian cuisine. They may also work well in other cooking methods, particularly as a seasoning for various pizza and lasagna varieties. Because of its antibacterial, analgesic, antidiarrheal, carminative, and anthelmintic qualities, this plant has a special place in traditional and folk medicine. Folk and traditional medicine frequently uses a variety of herbal products, including decoction, scented water, and essential oil. Many advantageous qualities, such as antinociceptive, antioxidant, antidiabetic, and anti-inflammatory activities, are demonstrated by contemporary pharmacological research on ZM. The Iranian pharmaceutical market offers this plant in several pharmacological forms, including syrups, oral drops, soft capsules, and vaginal creams, based on these properties. The pharmacological characteristics of ZM have currently been the subject of clinical trials. Stomatitis can have a variety of etiological reasons, such as immune system abnormalities, nutritional inadequacies, and infectious agents. Clinical research has shown that ZM is beneficial in reducing the symptoms of denture stomatitis and aphthous stomatitis, two different forms of stomatitis.

Although there are not currently authentic studies about the benefits of ZM for treating irritable bowel syndrome, some companies have introduced a commercial product called Gastrolit, which contains ZM essential oil in soft capsules and oral drop formulations. Gastrolit can help reduce the symptoms of irritable bowel syndrome. The impact of ZM extract on treating and preventing experimental inflammatory bowel disease in mice that were brought on by intrarectal acetic acid injection was examined in some studies. For comparison, prednisolone was utilized as the reference drug. Following ZM treatment, macroscopic, and microscopic character score values were much lower and were comparable to those of prednisolone. ZM exhibited an antioxidant effect. The *in vitro* research on the susceptibility of specific bacteria has provided researchers with the only information currently available regarding the potential benefits of ZM on intestinal infections. Many animal-based investigations have demonstrated the hepatoprotective action of ZM against a variety of toxic substances, such as paracetamol, oxidative stress generated by cisplatin, long-term administration of albendazole, cyclophosphamide, and CCl_4. While the herb is frequently used as a condiment in various food recipes, the majority of studies have concentrated on the administration of the plant extract or essential oil for a relatively short period.

5.4. The Promise of Cocoa

In addition to being one of the most valued ingredients due to its distinct flavor and aroma, cocoa is an interesting food since it is a rich source of bioactive components (Soares and Oliveira, 2022). The *Theobroma cacao* L. tree (fruit), which grows only in humid tropical areas, is used to make cocoa. After being harvested, cocoa fruits go through a fermentation process before drying. The dried cocoa nibs are roasted and crushed to make cocoa powder, cocoa butter, and cocoa liquor. Alkali is a common treatment used with cocoa powder to increase its solubility, darken its color, and neutralize its acidity. Due to its potential to stop chronic diseases like diabetes, cancer, obesity, neurological, and cardiovascular disorders, and aging, cocoa consumption has attracted attention in recent years. Consuming cocoa has the potential to alter both the intestinal gut-associated lymphoid tissue (GALT) and the gut microbiota. Certain intestinal bacteria and their functions, as well as the presence and functionality of immune cells in various GALT compartments, have all been demonstrated to be impacted by certain bioactive substances found in cocoa (Figure 5.2).

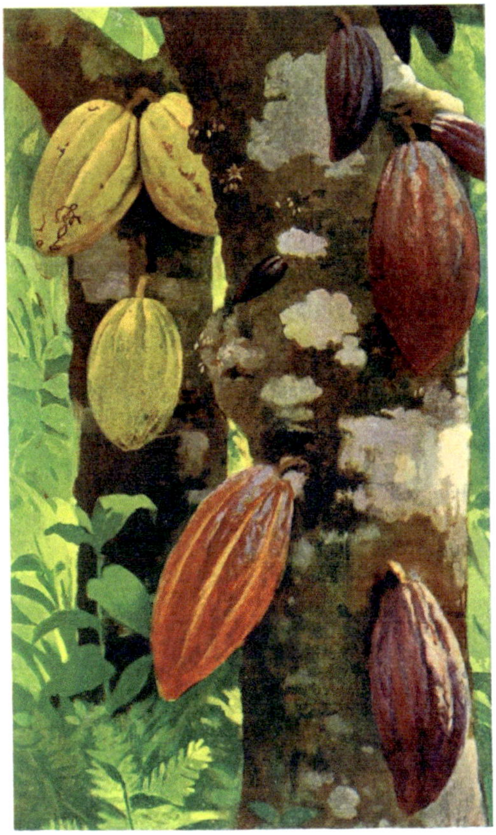

Figure 5.2. *Cocoa.*

Source: https://upload.wikimedia.org/wikipedia/commons/4/4a/Cacao_pods_-_Project_Gutenberg_eText_16035.jpg, Creative Commons License.

These qualities provide insights into the potential roles that cocoa may play in gastrointestinal disorders like intestinal inflammation and food allergies as a nutraceutical element. Water, proteins, fats, minerals, starch, pentosans, cellulose, sucrose, polyphenols, and alkaloids are present in fresh cocoa beans. The qualities of cocoa are attributed to theobromine, caffeine, nitrogen, and phenolic chemicals. Storage proteins like albumins, globulins, prolamins, and glutelins make up most of the protein content of cocoa. The polypeptide in cocoa beans is albumin, whereas globulins make up 43% of the total protein content. Globulins experience significant proteolysis during fermentation. Cocoa is composed of triacylglycerols, diacylglycerols, monoacylglycerols, polar lipids, and free fatty acids. Saturated and monounsaturated fatty acids make up most of the fat in cocoa butter, with some polyunsaturated linoleic.

Among the beneficial bioactive elements of cocoa that contribute to its antioxidant qualities are polyphenolic chemicals. The fruit ages and these substances build up within the cocoa bean. During this stage, the cocoa phenolic content is influenced by diverse factors including genetics, soil properties, sunlight, and rainfall, and harvesting timing. Other processing techniques that affect the amount of phenols in cocoa are fermentation, drying, alkalization, roasting, grinding, and conching. Of the phenolic chemicals present in cocoa, flavonoids are prevalent. These bioactive substances are made up of proanthocyanidins, anthocyanins, and monomers, such as catechin and epicatechin. In cocoa, the amounts of catechin and epicatechin vary. Subunits of epicatechin provide the basis for anthocyanins and procyanidins. Cyanidins-3-α-L-arabinoside and cyanidin-3-β-D-galactoside are the main types of anthocyanins. The majority of proanthocyanidins are flavan-3,4-diols, which have epicatechin as their primary subunit and are attached to dimers, trimers, or oligomers. Cocoa also has dietary fiber, which is composed of complex carbohydrates like cellulose, pectic components, and hemicellulose. Depending on the growth environment, cocoa, and chocolate may include substantial levels of minerals like magnesium, copper, potassium, and iron. Over 80% of the mass of cacao pods is made up of byproducts from the cocoa industry, such as the pulp, hull, husk, and shell (Rojo-Poveda et al., 2020). These by-products are becoming popular as animal feed because they are also high in bioactive compounds. Cocoa husks, when used in pig diet, have been demonstrated to positively impact certain health indices without adversely affecting productive routines. Several studies have reported the promoting or inhibiting effect of a cocoa-containing diet on specific intestinal microbiota microorganisms, despite the antibacterial activity of cocoa polyphenol extracts. Certain substances included in cocoa can enter the colon, and after making their way through the small and large intestines, they can have an impact on the microbiota of the gut. The impact of fiber and cocoa polyphenols on gut flora has been the subject of many studies. Apart from the direct impact of consuming cocoa on the growth of specific bacterial phylum, family, order, genus, or species, intestinal bacteria also play a role in the metabolism of the bioactive compounds found in cocoa, thereby establishing a mutual relationship between microbiota and diet. Preclinical research on rats using a diet supplemented with 10% w/w cocoa powder showed that the effects of cocoa on the gut varied according to the age of the animals and the duration of the nutritional intervention. Three weeks of a cocoa diet reduced the numbers of Bifidobacterium, Staphylococcus, and Streptococcus groups in young rats. Consumption of cocoa led to increased levels of *Eubacterium rectale*, *Clostridium coccoides*, and Bacteroides. The amount of the *Clostridium histolyticum subgroup*, the Bacteroides and Staphylococcus genera, and their proportion in the feces was significantly reduced after a prolonged dietary intervention lasting six weeks.

5.5. Bioactive Compounds in Cocoa

Several research studies attempted to determine the precise function of each of the bioactive components found in cocoa, polyphenols, fiber, and methylxanthines, in the gut microbiota. Studies conducted *in vitro*, preclinical, and even in humans have shown that the effects of cocoa on the gut microbiota may be attributed to cocoa polyphenols and their metabolites derived from microbes. In addition to their direct effects on intestinal microbiota and the excretion of part of unabsorbed flavanols into the stool, cocoa polyphenols can be metabolized by gut bacteria into simpler metabolites such as phenylpropionic, phenylacetic, and benzoic acid derivatives, which increases their bioavailability and creates new compounds that are more bioactive than the original forms found in food. Following intestine microbial action, some of the cocoa metabolites may enter the bloodstream, where they are primarily broken down by liver phase-II enzymes and then excreted in urine. Animals fed cocoa produce metabolites in their urine, some of which are produced by the gut microbiota (Sorrenti et al., 2020). Examples of these metabolites include hippurate and 2-hydroxyisobutyrate or 2-HIB, 4-hydroxypropionic acid or 4-HPA, phenylacetylglycine or PAG, and indole-3-acetic acid or IAA. These metabolites can be derived from the polyphenols and procyanidins found in cocoa, as well as from the amino acids tyrosine, phenylalanine, and tryptophan, or from the monoamines found in cocoa, as well as from the polyphenols and procyanidins. After consuming cocoa, urine has been found to contain microbially derived flavanol metabolites, such as 4-hydroxy-5-(3,4-dihydroxyphenyl) valeric acid and 5-(3,4-dihydroxyphenyl)-valerolactone. These findings show that intestinal microbiota plays a role in the metabolism of the cocoa compounds found in urine. There is a relationship between the effects of cocoa on rat gut microbiota and their urine metabolic profile following consumption. The proportion of the Streptococcus genus and the excretion of epicatechin and 4-hydroxypropionic acid in urine were found to be inversely correlated. A negative association (-ve) was observed between the Firmicutes to Bacteroidetes and the metabolites obtained from cocoa. These findings support the impact of cocoa polyphenols on gut microbes. After rats were fed a diet rich in cocoa, there was a lower excretion of N-methylnicotinamide or NMND, 3-indoxyl sulfate or 3-IS, and pseudouridine. This suggests a shift in the composition and functionality of the gut microbiota toward a less-oxidative profile. Because cocoa contains dietary fiber, it does not hydrolyze or break down in the stomach or small intestine and instead reaches the colon. The colonic microbiota can then use this fiber to convert it into oligosaccharides, which is how SCFA is formed. The dietary fiber may also indirectly affect the synthesis of SCFAs by changing the makeup of the gut microbiota.

5.6. Research on Cocoa Fiber

A cocoa fiber diet with nearly no polyphenols has been used to compare the contribution of cocoa fiber to the effects of natural cocoa on gut microbiota and SCFA production. A diet high in cocoa fiber had effects on *Bacteroides* spp. that were similar to those of natural cocoa, but it also increased the numbers of Bifidobacterium spp. and *Lactobacillus* spp. in rat feces. This suggests that the diet had prebiotic qualities. After four weeks of dietary intervention, the levels of Staphylococcus, Streptococcus, and *C. histolitycum* or *Clostridium perfringens* were higher in the cocoa fiber diet than in the cocoa diet. As a result of these modifications, the Firmicutes/Bacteroidetes ratio increased, which is not consistent with the results of a cocoa diet. However, feeding pigs a diet rich in fiber and polyphenols for three weeks had the tendency to lower the Firmicutes/Bacteroidetes ratio. This was because the intestinal populations of the Firmicutes group and the Bacteroides–Prevotella group (Bacteroidetes) decreased while the former increased. In the cocoa husk fed to pigs, Bifidobacterium did not exhibit any alterations. The urine metabolic profile of animals fed cocoa fiber has been assessed and compared with that of animals fed cocoa. Rats given cocoa fiber without polyphenols excreted less cocoa, catechin, and methylxanthine compounds in their urine than did the animals fed cocoa. Nevertheless, compared to the animals fed cocoa, it also led to the elimination of food derivatives like sucrose and glucose, acetone, citrate, 2-oxoglutarate, NMND, α-ketoisocaproate and β-hydroxy-β-methylbutyrate, and 3-IS. In young rats, the pattern of SCFA synthesis was likewise altered by cocoa fiber. A three-week cocoa fiber intake raised the concentration of total SCFA in the cecal and fecal contents due to an increase in all three main SCFA, i.e., acetic, propionic, and butyric acids. This was not the case for the animals fed cocoa, whose feces only showed an increase in butyric acid. Both diets based on cocoa and cocoa fiber acidified the pH of the cecum and feces in a similar manner, despite the fact that different SCFA profiles were found (Disca et al., 2024).

In addition to fiber and polyphenols, chocolate includes alkaloids like theobromine and caffeine whose impacts on the gut flora have also been studied. It is well known that theobromine enters the gut, where the microbiota can metabolize it. Theobromine alone was also able to lessen the presence of the Clostridium and Bacteroidaceae-Prevotellaceae groups, like the modifications brought about by a cocoa diet. However, utilizing fluorescence *in situ* hybridization in conjunction with flow cytometry, methylxanthine consumption alone decreased the counts of total bacteria in the feces, specifically lowering the counts of *E. coli*, *Bifidobacterium* spp., *Streptococcus* spp., and *C. histolyticum*–C. *perfringens*. As a result, theobromine consumption decreased the number of Firmicutes in feces without having a major impact on the ratio of Firmicutes to Bacteroids. Theobromine intake increased the proportion of certain members of the Firmicutes, Proteobacteria, and Tenericutes phyla, but did not affect the total counts of the Bacteroidetes and Firmicutes phyla, according to a metagenomic approach. The use of theobromine led to the removal of the Prevotella genus, but the consumption of cocoa enhanced it.

The amount of fiber in cocoa affects microbiota to some extent, but the presence of polyphenols and theobromine plays a significant role in enhancing, counteracting, or enhancing the effects of the fiber. In addition to the benefits that cocoa compounds provide for the intestinal microbiota, it has been shown that consuming cocoa can affect the GALT and the intestinal epithelium; these effects may be partially explained by the connection between cocoa and the intestinal microbiota. *In vivo* investigations have been performed to examine the GALT and its immune cell composition. The majority of these investigations were conducted on rodents due to the ability to extract and examine specific GALT cells. The major portion of the immune system is found in the intestine, which serves as the first line of defense against infections. One of the most significant functions of the GALT is the synthesis and secretion of immunoglobulin A (IgA), which offers defense against microorganisms. The distribution and function of the lymphoid intestinal structures determine their classification. Peyer's patches or PP and mesenteric lymph nodes (MLN) are examples of organized lymphoid tissues that serve as inductive sites for intestinal immune responses (Spahn et al., 2002). The lymphocytes from the epithelium (intraepithelial lymphocytes or IEL) and those positioned in the lamina propria (LPL), which take part in the intestine effector immunological responses, combine to produce the diffuse lymphoid tissues. The protection and homeostasis of the intestine are facilitated by each of these structures and cells. The function of cocoa and its polyphenolic extract on the colon may be determined using *in vitro* research conducted on the human cancer cell line called Caco-2, a model of the intestinal epithelial layer. The expression of ferritin heavy polypeptide 1 was upregulated in Caco-2 cells cultured with a cocoa extract for 24 hours, while the expression of mitogen-activated protein kinase 1, multidrug resistance-associated protein 1, and signal transducer & activator of transcription (STAT) 1 was downregulated. It has been observed that a cocoa polyphenolic extract may have an effect on intestinal inflammation in the model by inhibiting the formation of prostaglandin E2 in Caco-2 cells. According to these findings, interleukin (IL) 8 release was decreased in Caco-2 cells after pretreatment with 10 mg/mL cocoa polyphenolic extract for 20 hours. This was done after the cells had been stimulated with tumor necrosis factor (TNF) α for 24 hours. The cyclooxygenase (COX) 2 and inducible nitric oxide synthase (iNOS), two inflammatory enzymes, had lower protein levels in such cocoa-containing environments.

5.7. Polyphenols in Cocoa

The primary polyphenols of cocoa, (+)-catechin, (−)-epicatechin, and procyanidin B2 have been found, indicating a paracellular pathway of transport and its potential impact on impairing tight junction function. The rat intestinal immune system is impacted by eating a diet containing 10% (w/w) cocoa, which reduces the amount of intestinal IgA produced. When young rats mature, their intestinal IgA level rises; this growing trend was circumvented by feeding them a diet that contained 10% cocoa. In young, healthy Lewis rats, the IgA-attenuating effect can be seen as soon as 4 days after cocoa administration. The effect on intestinal IgA was not statistically significant at lower chocolate doses examined. Lower intestinal IgA gene expression and a decreased percentage of IgA+ cells in the lamina propria correlated with the decline in intestinal IgA protein levels. While the exact process by which cocoa produces this action is still unknown, some theories have been put forth. As of now, consumption of cocoa downregulated the expression of genes involved in the intestinal migration of lymphocytes, such as the retinoic acid receptors α and β, which are both involved in the retinoic acid IgA isotype switching, and the gut homing receptor, and

CC chemokine receptor 9. The use of cocoa reduced the expression of genes related to the synthesis of IgA, including transforming growth factor β, which are involved in the activation and differentiation of B lymphocytes. However, a decrease in the percentage of intraepithelial cells expressing Toll-like receptor, a receptor linked to the release of cytokines involved in the recruitment and differentiation of IgA+ B cells, may also be connected to the attenuating effect on intestinal IgA. It has been demonstrated in rats that diets containing cocoa polyphenols also attenuated the fecal IgA concentration, indicating the role of each cocoa component in the attenuating action on intestinal IgA. There was an inverse relationship between the amount of epicatechin derivatives in urine and the fecal IgA concentration.

On the other hand, there was no dose-response effect observed in relation to the amount of polyphenols, which implies that other cocoa chemicals may possibly impact IgA. Thus, the impact of natural cocoa in rats and the effect of cocoa fiber consumption on intestinal IgA were compared. Investigation revealed that while IgA production was reduced in other mucosal compartments, a diet high in cocoa fiber alone improved IgA synthesis in MLN. This also mitigated the intestinal IgA levels. The mechanisms generated by the ingestion of cocoa fiber did not align with those caused by natural cocoa, indicating that fiber was not the primary factor responsible for the attenuating effect of cocoa on intestinal IgA.

By comparing the effects of a diet high in cocoa and one with the same quantity of theobromine as the first diet, the role of the major methylxanthine in cocoa was determined. These studies demonstrate that theobromine has the same effect on intestinal IgA as cocoa. This result is supported by the observation that there is an inverse relationship between the amount of methylxanthine derivatives in urine and the fecal IgA concentration. It appears that theobromine content was primarily responsible for the alterations in intestinal immunoglobulin secretion, although catechins may also have an impact.

5.8. Gut Microbiota and Cocoa

Some alterations in the gut microbiota have been linked to the impact on intestinal IgA. A decrease in the proportion of IgA-coated bacteria in feces was consistent with the impact of a 10% cocoa diet on intestinal IgA concentration. This was also noted following the consumption of theobromine. Consuming diets with increased levels of cocoa polyphenol, however, did not have an appropriate impact. The quantity of fecal *Lactobacillus, Bifidobacterium,* and *Streptococcus* genera was positively connected with the fraction of IgA-coated bacteria (DuPont et al., 2023). There was a correlation between a drop in the numbers of Streptococcus genera and the low intestine IgA content caused by a chocolate diet. There was a positive link observed between intestinal IgA levels and the *Proteobacteria phylum*, and these immunoglobulins and the alterations in the microbiota of animals fed cocoa.

5.9. The Effect of Cocoa on Immunological Reactions

IgA levels could potentially be indicative of shifts in the lymphoid cell distribution inside the gut. As demonstrated in rats, cocoa consumption also affects the immune cells in the GALT effector sites. Regarding inductive sites, a 10% cocoa diet raised the percentage of T-cell receptor γδ+ and natural killer (NK) cells in

MLN. TCRγδ+ cells were prevalent because of a cluster of differentiation (CD) 8αα+ cells, which have an intestinal phenotype and may have migrated from the epithelia. The percentage of NK and TCRγδ+ cells in the PP was similarly higher when a diet containing 10% cocoa was consumed. Consequently, a cocoa diet boosts intestinal immunity by increasing the presence of these innate immune-related cells, even while it has a weakening effect on intestinal IgA. The distribution of TCRαβ+ subsets was altered in both MLN and PP by the cocoa dietary intervention, resulting in a decline in the percentage of T helper (Th) cells. Given that there may have been less intestinal B-cell activation when the Th cell fraction dropped, this result could help to partially explain the lower intestinal IgA synthesis. A 10% cocoa diet also increased the proportion of regulatory cells like CD^{25+} and CD^{103+} cells in these lymphoid tissues, while decreasing the proportion of cells expressing CD62L (Camps-Bossacoma et al., 2017). This difference may suggest that fewer lymphocytes were able to reach these tissues.

Rats that consumed cocoa also had a higher proportion of TCRγδ+ lymphocytes and NK cells in IEL in the effector sites of the GALT, similar to what happened in the inductive sites of the GALT. This observation implies that rats fed with cocoa had improved gut immunity. However, the intervention with cocoa did not alter the cellular types found in the lamina propria. Some research studies were aimed at identifying the cocoa chemicals that were causing these alterations in the composition of lymphocytes in the gut. The consumption of cocoa with a larger portion of polyphenols did not cause the changes in MLN and PP that were observed, and there is no proof that cocoa fiber has any effect. However, the GALT had comparable alterations when consuming the same quantity of theobromine as the cocoa diet, indicating that it is similarly crucial for intestinal immunity. Several preclinical investigations have been carried out to examine the impact of cocoa consumption on gastrointestinal tract pathologies. It is interesting to note how cocoa affects inflammatory bowel disease (IBD) models. It has been claimed that cocoa polyphenols prevent ulcerative colitis in a mouse model of the disease caused by ingestion of dextran sulfate sodium (DSS). The consumption of a 5% cocoa-enriched diet for five weeks in a rat model of DSS did not alter the colon DSS shortening, but it did lessen the colon cell infiltration and goblet cell loss. The reduction in colon iNOS activity and serum TNF-α levels demonstrated the anti-inflammatory qualities of cocoa.

Although certain inflammatory reactions could not be prevented, the published data indicate that cocoa intervention at the investigated dosages decreased the oxidative stress associated with colitis. Cocoa function in IBD is reinforced by its preventive effect on colitis linked to cancer through diet. Azoxymethane (AOM) and DSS are administered, and the result is a model with cancer linked to colitis. Certain alterations in the AOM/DSS-treated mice were avoided by a 10% cocoa diet, including the increase in colonic malondialdehyde levels, the expression of the COX-2 and iNOS genes, and the fall in enzymatic antioxidants. A diet high in 10% cocoa prevented colon damage. Feeding 5% and 10% cocoa inhibited the colon macrophage infiltration while also reducing the gene expression of TNF-α, IL-1β, IL-6, and IL-17 in a dose-dependent manner. Preclinical research suggests that eating chocolate could be helpful as an additional IBD treatment. Still, additional research on dose needs to be done in addition to clinical trials. In addition to IBD, cocoa consumption has been shown to protect against food allergies due to its immunoregulatory properties. A food allergy is an aberrant immunological response that is brought on by a harmless food protein and manifests as a range of symptoms. In particular, the food antigen triggers an immune response, leading to the generation of IgE, which then acts on mast cells to produce the symptoms of allergies. Preclinical research has demonstrated how chocolate can prevent food allergies from developing. This was initially reported in an allergy model in which Brown Norway rats were injected with ovalbumin (OVA), alum, and Bordetella pertussis toxin, followed by an oral OVA treatment. According to preclinical research on systemic allergy, the consumption of a 10% cocoa-enriched diet completely inhibited the generation of anti-OVA IgE and other antibodies linked to Th2 responses (Abril-Gil et al., 2012). Due to the attenuating action of cocoa on intestinal IgA, the food allergy caused a rise in intestine anti-OVA IgA, which was prevented by the cocoa diet. The reduction in the gene expression of the rat mast cell mucosal protease (RMCP-II), which is produced by the same cells in the small intestine, and the high-affinity IgE receptor on mast cells were the mechanisms behind the antiallergic effects of cocoa. Consuming cocoa also reduced the production of Th1-related cytokines like IL-1α, IL-1β, and interferon γ generated by MLN and prevented an increase in Th2-related cytokines like IL-5 and IL-13. Feeding on cocoa affected the spleen synthesis of IL-6 and IL-13 while weakening that of IL-4 and the systemic immune system.

5.10. Anti-Anaphylactic Responses and Other Impacts of Cocoa

The role of cocoa consumption in an anaphylactic response following an oral exposure was also assessed. Eating cocoa did not prevent the allergy from causing changes in body temperature, motor activity, intestinal permeability, or serum RMCP-II levels, but it did aid in the elevated hematocrit recovery. In Lewis rats, an oral immunological sensitization to OVA was likewise prevented by a cocoa diet. Consuming cocoa powder reduced the amount of serum anti-OVA antibodies produced, primarily due to the absence of anti-OVA IgG1, IgG2b, and IgM, and it elevated the amount of IL-10 in the intestines, which may be connected to the tolerogenic properties of cocoa. The cocoa diet reduced the cytokine that inhibits oral tolerance, IL-17α, and its gene expression in MLN. In small intestine samples from the oral sensitization model, consumption of cocoa similarly decreased the expression of the dendritic cell markers CD11b and CD11c. Its expression was elevated in MLN, indicating that it migrated to this lymphoid compartment to support oral tolerance. Alterations in the gut flora may also be connected to cocoa's ability to prevent food allergies. Orally sensitized rats were given either normal or cocoa-enriched foods. The results of a metagenomic research showed that the cocoa diet caused the development of the Streptophyta order and increased abundance of *Bacteroides uniformis*. A cocoa diet on oral sensitive rats caused *Prevotella copri* to appear and the Prevotella genus to be more abundant; these effects were also shown in healthy volunteers who drank red wine polyphenols. Cocoa significantly increased the amount of *Lactobacillus reuteri*, a bacterial species known to affect the immunological responses in the intestines. Despite these modifications, it is challenging to link the tolerogenic impact of the chocolate diet to a specific bacterium, and more research is required to comprehend the connection between gut microbiota and food allergies.

5.11. Synbiotics

Synbiotics are combinations of probiotics and prebiotics, growth promoters for probiotics, which promote the survival of live microbial dietary supplements in the gastrointestinal or GI tract and have a positive effect on the host. Prebiotics have a large effect on host health by either increasing the generation of metabolites or selectively boosting the growth of probiotics and activating the metabolism of health-promoting bacteria. Probiotic strains-fortified foods and fermented dairy products typically contain live probiotic cultures, but freeze-dried probiotics can also be obtained commercially in the form of pills, capsules, powders, or sachets. Probiotic strains that have been documented include *Saccharomyces cerevisiae*, *Bacillus coagulans*, and *L. reuteri* (Fijan, 2014). Reducing bacteriophage contamination and creating starting strains resistant to phages are top priorities for industrial technologists and researchers alike. Probiotic strains, particularly Lactobacillus, have a variety of general characteristics, such as the capacity to regulate both innate and acquired immunity and to preserve the gut epithelium. They also possess antimicrobial properties against enteric pathogens through the secretion of hydrogen peroxide, organic acids, and antimicrobial polypeptides. These unique qualities are related to their roles in the treatment and prevention of diarrhea and (chronic) intestinal infections. This bacterial strategy aims to prevent and exclude the growth of harmful bacteria by populating all possible gut niches with beneficial bacteria. The production of antimicrobial agents like lactic acids, H_2O_2, and bacteriocins, the synthesis of SCFAs, the improvement of the immune system, the prevention of colonization and adhesion, and the modification of mucosal barrier functions are just a few of the beneficial qualities linked to the ability to combat foodborne disease. They have been shown to have positive effects on human digestion, reduce inflammation, inhibit the growth of cancer, aid in absorption, and lower cholesterol. It has been discovered that Lactobacillus and Bifidobacterium both improve colonization resistance, which helps them compete with intestinal bacterial infections. Enterococcus faecium, probiotic bifidobacteria, and nonpathogenic beneficial *E. coli* strains reduced the generation of Shiga toxin, prevented pathogenic EHEC growth, and shielded mice against EHEC infection. By competitive exclusion and displacement, several Lactobacillus strains, such as L. acidophilus, L. casei, L. fermentum, and L. rhamnosus, could attach themselves to host intestinal cells with efficiency and reduce the intestinal and extraintestinal dissemination of EHEC, Salmonella, *C. jejuni*, and *V. parahaemolyticus*. The administration of many probiotic strains in combination may have a synergistic effect on lowering *Shigella sonnei*, *Pseudomonas aeruginosa*, Salmonella, *Staphylococcus aureus*, and *Proteus mirabilis*. Probiotics like *Lactobacillus paracasei* have also been demonstrated to upregulate helper T cells and the production of antibodies, downregulate proinflammatory cytokines, and upregulate dendritic cells. These actions have been linked to improved or reversed gut integrity and protection against enteric bacterial pathogens, particularly Salmonella.

5.12. Prebiotics

Prebiotics are commonly known to contain oligosaccharides, lactulose, and inulin (Davani-Davari et al., 2019). They are characterized by being resistant to digestion enzymes in the human stomach and fermentable by colonic bacteria. A number of preliminary studies have shown that a number of bifidogenic prebiotics may supply native microflora that limits nutrients and energy for fermentation. These microflorae may do this by either releasing antimicrobial byproducts as a competitive advantage to drive out pathogenic bacteria or by producing vitamins, SCFAs, and antioxidants to modify the composition of intestinal microflora. In addition to these benefits, studies have shown that prebiotics may also stimulate the absorption of minerals, improve the efficiency of the immune system, and lower the risk of colon cancer. In the past years, researchers have been developing new genetically recombinant probiotics that offer even more benefits, like increased mucosal and intestinal colonization capacity, increased resistance to bacteriophage, gastric acid, and bile salts for GI tract survival, longer colonization time, increased competition with enteric pathogens, and increased expression of target antimicrobial molecules against pathogens. There are several bioengineering techniques that could be used to accomplish these goals. Initially, the surface of probiotic strains may express toxin-specific host cell receptors, which would enable them to interact competitively with deadly toxins released by enteric pathogens. To create a competitive environment for particular pathogen colonization, adhesions, and other important components of intestinal pathogen secretory systems could be cloned and produced on probiotic strains. Probiotic strains may disrupt the pathogenic quorum-sensing system and inhibit the target pathogen virulence gene expression by imitating the expression of virulence genes from enteric bacteria. The use of probiotic bacteria expressing heterologous antigens may elicit immunological reactions (cytokines), help reduce intestinal inflammation, and offer cytoprotection.

We need to understand the role of probiotics in preventing the colonization of enteric bacterial pathogens in the human gut and intestine, as well as their ability to secrete antimicrobial components, compete with pathogens for nutrient uptake, and block host cell receptors to inhibit pathogen growth and eliminate them. Enteric bacterial infections cannot infiltrate the GI tract because probiotics maintain a low pH environment there. Probiotics that work well are those that can tolerate and break down in the acidic environment of the stomach flora. Probiotics that thrive in low pH conditions include those in the Lactobacillus genus. The acidic environment may make some intestinal bacterial pathogens incapable of surviving, giving probiotics a significant competitive advantage. Intestinal bacterial pathogens like streptococci can withstand a cytoplasmic pH of approximately 5.7–7.6, but lactobacilli can withstand more acidic environments with a pH of about 4.4. Probiotic strains help bacteria maintain pH homeostasis because they can sustain an alkaline internal pH in comparison to the cytoplasmic pH of the internal epithelial cell (IEC). Probiotics have an edge over enteric infections because they produce organic acids that alter the gut microbiota. *Lactobacilli*, for example, metabolize glucose to produce lactic acid (lower the pH of the gut). This results in a lactic acid inhibitory action that targets *Salmonella enterica* and enteropathogenic *E. coli* (EPEC), two Gram-negative bacteria. These intestinal pathogens are unable to thrive in such an environment due to the competitive advantage of the probiotic strain. However, other enteric bacterial pathogens, including *Helicobacter pylori*, can also change the environment of the stomach.

5.13. Lactic Acid Bacteria

Because it can raise intracellular pH and acidify the cytoplasm, lactic acid produced by lactic acid bacteria, including Lactobacilli, is an important antibacterial agent. To break the proton-motive force, lactic acid must first enter the cell and subsequently dissociate into lactate within the cell. For probiotic strains to maintain a healthy internal pH balance, protons must be removed from the cytoplasm by H^+-ATPases. Enteric bacterial pathogens, like *Yersinia enterocolitica* (Figure 5.3) and *E. coli* M23, develop at a speed that is inversely proportional to the concentration of undissociated lactic acid, which lowers the pH inside IECs.

Enteric pathogen growth is inhibited if the pH is lowered to a specific level. The gut mucosa is where probiotic microorganisms and the host mostly interact. Probiotics compete with enteric pathogens for adhesion sites at the intestinal epithelial barrier in addition to the competition for nutrition. To stop harmful bacteria from attaching to the intestinal mucosa, which is mainly made up of mucins, probiotic strains have improved adherence to it. Certain probiotic strains generate proteins that enable mucosal layer surface attachment. *L. reuteri* produces a mucus-binding protein that facilitates the probiotic strain's adherence to the intestinal mucosa. Probiotics continue to colonize the gut because of their proteins, which are involved in the competitive exclusion of intestinal pathogens. To stop pathogen-dominant organisms from entering the host, probiotics also attach to host glycoprotein or host glycolipid adhesion receptors. Enteric infections primarily target the competition of adherence of the epithelial sites for entry (Sousa et al., 2005). For instance, *L. johnsonii* interacts with a glycolipid receptor on gangliotetraosylceramide to inhibit the binding of enteropathogenic bacteria, including EPEC. EPEC utilizes this host glycolipid receptor as a target host adhesion ligand. To promote defense against enteric pathogens, many probiotics specifically bind to Toll-like receptors (TLRs) on intestinal epithelial cells (IECs) to effectively inhibit adhesion sites where the pathogens can adhere. Following activation, TLRs react to patterns of molecules linked to pathogens. When TLRs are activated, important signaling pathways like the NF-κB and MAPK pathways are influenced, which permits an inflammatory response. Depending on which TLRs are activated, different outcomes may occur. For example, cytokine production can be increased by activating TLR2. Because TLR2 naturally recognizes peptidoglycan, which is abundant in Gram-positive bacteria like Lactobacillus strains, it binds to probiotics. Enteric pathogens are Gram-negative bacteria that have reduced peptidoglycan levels. This makes it harder for them to bind to TLR2 and withstand probiotics. Examples of these pathogens are *Salmonella enterica* and EPEC. More TLR2 expression in response to specific probiotic strains led to a rise in IL-10 secretion, which in turn reduced the inflammatory response. TLR9 activation occurs via either the basolateral or apical surface. While basolateral TLR9 degrades IκBα and activates the NF-κB pathway, apical TLR9 promotes the cytoplasmic accumulation of ubiquitinated IκB and inhibits the NF-κB system. By sticking to the mucosal layer and receptors, certain probiotic bacteria advance the colonization of the gut and successfully block the adherence of enteric pathogens.

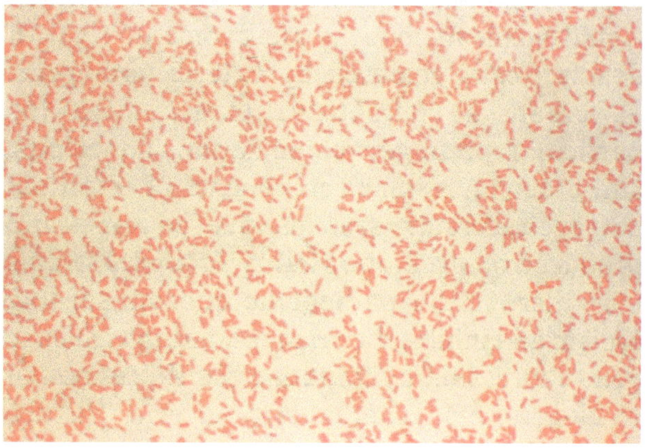

Figure 5.3. *Yersinia enterocolitica.*

Source: https://upload.wikimedia.org/wikipedia/commons/c/c9/Yersinia_enterocolitica_gram.jpg, Creative Commons License.

5.14. Other Mechanisms of Lactic Acid Bacteria

The intestinal epithelium barrier is the first line of protection that needs to be preserved since it stimulates host resistance. Probiotics work to modulate inflammation by either activating or blocking the NF-κB pathway, which strengthens the epithelial barrier (Wan et al., 2016). Different probiotic strains in intestinal epithelial cells have distinct functions based on their ability to either stimulate or inhibit the NF-κB pathway. This enables a modification in the epithelial barrier inflammation. An ideal level of inflammation is necessary to preserve the epithelial barrier and keep enteric bacteria from colonizing. Probiotics, such as *Bifidobacterium lactis*, activate NF-κB pathways, which advance epithelial barrier inflammation by secreting more of the proinflammatory cytokine IL-6. Low inflammatory levels help to keep the epithelium barrier intact. Other probiotics, including *Lactobacillus fermentum*, block NF-κB pathways, which lessens proinflammatory cytokine release and thus epithelial barrier inflammation. Controlling the various probiotic strains permits the normal level of inflammation needed to maximize the function of the epithelial barrier. Probiotics control inflammation in order to prevent enteric infections. The main function of the NF-κB pathway is to regulate the epithelial barrier strength. MAPK pathways have the ability to completely activate this pathway. Increasing the synthesis of mucin and antimicrobial peptides, reducing IEC programmed cell death, and reducing the generation of tumor necrosis factor alpha (TNF-α) are strategies for strengthening the epithelial barrier. *L. rhamnosus* suppresses TNF-α to stop apoptosis brought on by cytokines. Probiotics have the ability to enhance mucin expression, which helps to maintain and protect the epithelial barrier in addition to improving adhesion. Heat shock proteins allow IECs to survive without undergoing programmed cell death. When IECs are under stress, heat shock proteins trigger transcriptional activation, enabling them to preserve tight connections between IECs and strengthen the epithelial barrier. *L. rhamnosus* increases the mRNA levels of particular heat shock proteins by transcriptionally activating MAPK. The inhibition of proinflammatory cytokine TNF-α production keeps epithelial barriers from leaking and keeps them intact.

5.15. Gels and Probiotics

The first technique involves the prebiotic giving the probiotics nourishment, which increases the probiotic's development and release of metabolic byproducts. The use of microencapsulation is the second technique. Probiotics are quickly broken down in the stomach before they can help the host in the small intestine, which is a significant drawback of probiotic administration. Prebiotics are highly indigestible, so researchers have made use of this property to create a gel capsule that will only break down in the lower gastrointestinal tract. The gel capsule breaks down in the small intestine, allowing the probiotics to begin colonizing in the intestinal epithelium. There is an indirect symbiotic impact from the third technique. Probiotics and prebiotics are supplements that are taken concurrently (Pandey et al., 2015). However, the pathogenic bacteria bind to the prebiotics and are eliminated before they have an opportunity to colonize the intestinal epithelium, allowing the probiotics to take over and colonize the GI system. While less is known about the mechanisms involved in humans, probiotics, and prebiotics have been shown to control disease predominantly in animal models. The different regulatory mechanisms are specific to the probiotics and prebiotics under investigation.

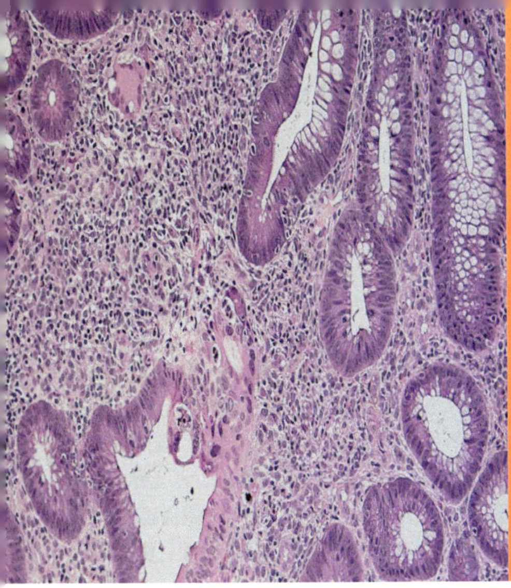

Chapter 6

MOLECULAR PATHOLOGY OF GI DISEASES

Contents

6.1. Introduction

The prevalence of gastrointestinal tract neoplastic disorders is constantly growing. The most common cause of morbidity is intestinal cancer. According to GLOBOCAN data from 2008, there are 3.8 million instances of GI malignancies annually, with 3.2 million deaths related to these cases (Kim et al., 2014). Over the past 40 years, a huge amount of resources has been used to better understand, prevent, and treat these diseases due to the unusually high number of patients who are affected. We now understand that gastrointestinal tract cancers vary widely in kind and are caused by intricate interactions between host and environmental variables. Normal mucosa may become precursor lesions, premalignant lesions, or even cancer as a result of this interaction. There are several basic characteristics that are shared by malignancies in different cell types and tissues. Neoplastic transformed cells are unable to react to signals that control their own differentiation, replication, migration, and death (apoptosis). Neoplasms can arise from any tissue in the body and in the GI tract. They can also cause extrinsic invasion or compression, the use of metabolic resources, and metastatic spreading to other parts of the body. Hence, tumors, whether benign or malignant, can have a significant impact on a patient's health. The current model of cancer biology, which describes carcinogenesis as a complex process requiring numerous sequential genetic alterations (mutations), was developed in response to the realization that cancer is a disease caused by gene mutations and that there is a biologically discernible, stepwise pattern leading to cancer. It was believed before the arrival of this idea that tumor growth and start were separate genetic and biological processes. Growing evidence that suggests cancers are clonal, originating from a single progenitor that has acquired the required mutations to undergo neoplastic transformation, has reinforced (strengthened) the multistep concept. At this point, it is thought that mutations happen randomly and that only very uncommon mutations can cause the silence of tumor suppressor pathways or the improper activation of growth promoters. These cells therefore have a distinct survival advantage over neighboring normal cells due to these uncommon mutations. These mutations are progressively acquired.

6.2. Genetic Mutations

It is believed that the number of genetic mutations needed for clonal proliferation and malignant transformation varies depending on the tissue under investigation, the gene combinations used, and the genetic makeup of the individual, including gene polymorphisms. According to current estimates, four to seven average necessary mutations are needed for most cancers. This presents a significant concern, especially for epithelial tissues that are in a state of constant turnover. Stem cells are the only cells that are kept long enough to accumulate three to seven mutations in important genes, even though mutations are thought to be primarily random occurrences. Thus, the idea that stem cells play a role in the development of cancer has been supported by many research studies. Some mutations can change population dynamics by causing some non-stem cells to acquire mutations that enhance survival or change migratory or differentiation patterns. Improper cell division and unregulated growth are caused by mutations in genes essential for cell proliferation, differentiation, and death. These mutations also make the cell more susceptible to subsequent mutations. These mutations can occur sporadically or be inherited. These mutations can be accelerated by exposure to a variety of environmental variables, such as carcinogens and long-term immune-compromising diseases. It was determined after many years of observation and research that long-term immune disorders are linked to cancer in several organ systems and tissues. It is possible that the gastrointestinal tract is especially susceptible to currently unknown causes. Each of the GI tract's primary organs is susceptible to one or more disease processes, which can lead to a chronic inflammatory condition. All of these processes, chemical, viral, bacterial, and genetic, have varying etiologies, but they are all known to raise the risk of cancer.

6.3. Pancreatitis

Patients with hereditary pancreatitis (Figure 6.1) provide an example of the link between long-term immune disorders and malignancy (Schneider and Whitcomb, 2002). Most kinds of hereditary pancreatitis are brought on by inherited mutations in the PRSS1 gene, which codes for cationic trypsinogen. Acute pancreatitis episodes are caused by these mutations, which increase trypsin stability or trypsinogen autoactivation. Not long after this hereditary disease was identified, it was discovered that high rates of pancreatic cancer also occurred in other family types. Only after 20 or more years of recurrent pancreatitis do pancreatic malignancies develop, indicating that persistent inflammation rather than the PRSS1 mutation is the source of the malignancy. Thus, this trend lends credibility to the theory that long-term exposure to fluoride can encourage pancreatic cancer. Ulcerative colitis (UC) is a recurrent, chronic inflammatory colon disease that has a strong correlation to the development of cancer. Persons with UC may have a cumulative cancer risk of up to 60%. The extent, length, and severity of the disease are now known to influence the risk of colon cancer in people with UC. Given that the yearly and cumulative occurrences of colon cancer in UC increase from 0.2% and 1.6%, respectively, after 10 years of disease to 1.2% and 18.4%, respectively, after 30 years of UC, disease duration is the established risk factor. The degree of the disease is another clinically significant component; pancolitis increases the risk of colon cancer by 20 times compared to rectum diseases. All of these relationships lend credibility to the concept that a long-term inflammatory process may aid in the development of cancer. It has been shown by epidemiological research looking at the relationship between the use of aspirin and other NSAIDs and the risk of cancer that regular users of these drugs have lower incidences of stomach, colon, and esophageal cancers. Meta-analyses have shown that patients with familial adenomatous polyposis (FAP), a genetic susceptibility to colon cancer, or those with stomach and esophageal malignancies may benefit from regular aspirin or NSAID use as a chemoprotective measure. A multitude of epidemiological, biological, and pharmacologic studies have demonstrated that the indoor environment plays a significant role in the development of many gastrointestinal malignancies in humans.

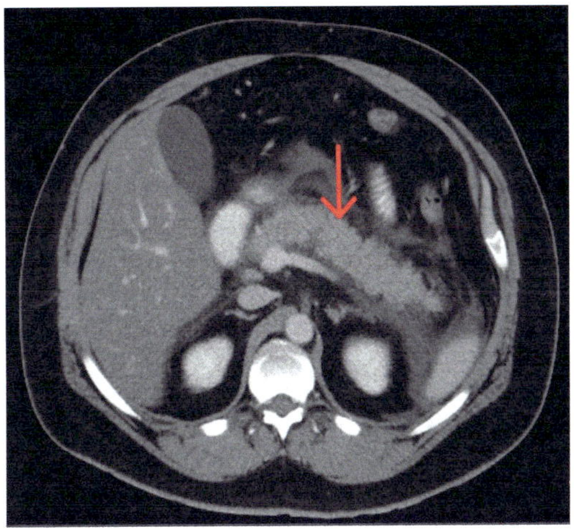

Figure 6.1. *Pancreatitis.*

Source: https://upload.wikimedia.org/wikipedia/commons/9/97/Pankreatitis_exsudativ_CT_axial.jpg, Creative Commons License.

6.4. Cancer Cell Features

Cancer cells develop a wide range of mutations. This has made it more difficult for researchers to create therapeutic methods that work and to comprehend the process mechanistically. Some researchers proposed a different model that identified six distinguishing characteristics that all tumors must have in order to be classified as successful cancer. These are: self-sufficiency (proliferative signals), insensitivity (antiproliferative signals), resistance to apoptosis, maintenance of telomeres, self-directed angiogenesis and the ability to invade tissues locally and spread to distant locations. The observation that genetic abnormalities could lead to increased functionality and unchecked cell division was initially recognized through the investigation of DNA viruses and retroviruses that were connected to malignancies in both humans and animals. These early investigations identified viral genes capable of causing neoplastic transformation. We can call these genes as oncogenes. Similar sequences were found in the human genome. These human genes are now referred to as proto-oncogenes, and other studies have shown that human cancers usually involve mutations in the regulators of these genes, which causes constitutive activation of the proto-oncogenes. 80 human protooncogenes have been identified since the discovery of the human oncogene HRAS (Tsuchida et al., 2016). Peptide growth factors, receptor, and non-receptor tyrosine kinases, signal transduction proteins connected to cell membranes, and nuclear transcription factors are the four main groups of proto-oncogenes. It has been discovered that each of them significantly affects differentiation, proliferation, and cell cycle control. In gastrointestinal malignancies, many proto-oncogenes can activate simultaneously, and tumor growth requires these genes' continuous activity. In addition to inhibiting tumor growth, disruption of these stimulatory signals may also cause cell death and apoptosis to be induced. As a result, it has been proposed that malignancies are oncogene-dependent, and researchers are currently investigating treatment approaches.

6.5. Oncogenes and Neoplasia

Neoplasia can arise as a result of several proto-oncogene mutation types. Persistently active proteins can be produced by gene rearrangements, point mutations, and insertion/deletion events that irreversibly change the structure of the gene product. Proto-oncogene regulatory domains are susceptible to disruption or inactivation by these similar mechanisms. Oncogene mRNA synthesis can also be elevated by mutations. Therefore, all of these mutations lead to either improper proto-oncogene expression or loss of proto-oncogene regulator function. Delays in differentiating, unchecked cell division, and proliferation are the outcomes. The arrangement of genes varies greatly between tissues and even within the same malignancy, even though many proto-oncogenes are usually activated simultaneously in transformed cells. Proto-oncogenes are frequently found in critical growth-signaling pathways in an epistatic succession. All of these mutations would have the same phenotypic result. The epithelial growth factor signaling cascade is one instance. This signaling pathway links EGF, the receptor EGFR, KRAS, JUN (c-jun), and MYC (c-myc) (Wee and Wang, 2017). Up to 90% of pancreatic cancers and 50% of colorectal cancers have KRAS mutations; however, esophageal tumors are far less likely to have these mutations. As a result, even though 90% of esophageal squamous cell carcinomas lack KRAS mutations, EGFR gene amplification causes these cancers to have elevated EGFR activity. A crucial characteristic of cancerous cells is the gain-of-function mutations in proto-oncogenes, which lead to self-sufficiency in cell division. Proto-oncogenes encourage cell division; however, tumor suppressor genes typically closely regulate this process. Research on retinoblastoma led to the identification of genes that closely regulate proliferation. There are two types of this uncommon pediatric retinal cancer: familial and sporadic retinal retinoblastoma. It was observed that the sporadic type was far less common than the familial form. There might be a genetic connection between these two uncommon disease forms. Researchers hypothesized that two mutations in the same gene were the cause of this disease. One of these mutations was inherited in the germline in the familial form of retinoblastoma, while the other mutation was acquired. The spontaneous type of the disease has a significantly lower incidence because both copies had to undergo mutation through somatic mechanisms.

6.6. Tumor Gene Targets

Tumor suppressor gene mutations are only loss-of-function occurrences. Similar to retinoblastoma, (Figure 6.2) the progression of neoplastic growth necessitates the biallelic inactivation of all tumor suppressors. The first allele in a germline disease caused by a mutation in a tumor suppressor has been made nonfunctional. Usually, allelic loss, often referred to as loss of heterozygosity (LOH), or epigenetic gene silencing, are used to inactivate the second allele. It has been demonstrated that promoter hypermethylation is crucial for the silence of several tumor suppressor genes. The loss of the second functional allele in a daughter cell during cell division, or LOH, is caused by nonreciprocal translocation. Finding areas of chromosomes sensitive to LOH and searching inside them for potential tumor suppressor genes has led to the discovery of several tumor suppressor genes. As transcription factors, adhesion proteins, cell surface receptors, intracellular signaling proteins, or apoptotic signaling proteins, tumor suppressor genes can perform a variety of functions. Responsible for controlling the cell cycle transition from the G1 to the S phase, RB (retinoblastoma gene) is an essential regulator. By attaching to many transcription factors in the E2F family and suppressing the expression of genes that these factors normally regulate, RB prevents the departure from G1. The normal S phase of DNA replication and nucleotide synthesis depends on these E2F target genes. Cyclin-dependent kinases (CDKs) phosphorylate RB, which reduces its binding affinity for certain transcription factors (Malumbres, 2014). This strictly regulates RB. Unrestricted cell division and unchecked advancement through the cell cycle are made possible by RB inactivation. Thus, altering RB function is a crucial stage in a lot of neoplastic processes. In gastrointestinal cancers, RB is not altered. However, several GI malignancies use different strategies to change RB function. Multiple mechanisms of RB suppression have been shown in human malignancies, including overexpression or stability of cyclin-dependent kinase (CDK) and silencing or mutation-mediated inhibition of CDK inhibitors (CDKIs), p21, p27, and p16. As potential new therapeutic targets, researchers are actively working to reconstruct the role of these CDKIs in cancers. P53 is another tumor suppressor that is commonly impacted in cancer. Up to 50% of human cancers are estimated to be caused by this gene product dysfunction. Since P53 was shown to cause neoplastic transformation in rat embryonic fibroblasts, it was first believed to encourage immortalization.

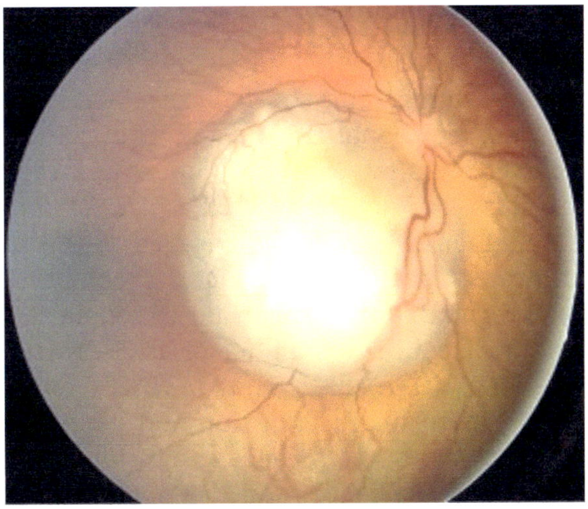

Figure 6.2. *Retinoblastoma.*

Source: https://upload.wikimedia.org/wikipedia/commons/3/3d/Fundus_retinoblastoma.jpg, Creative Commons License.

6.7. The Biology of P53

Significant investigation revealed that p53 is a transcription factor that is triggered by metabolic stresses, abnormal growth signals, and direct DNA damage. The DNA Damage Response (DDR) mechanism is triggered when DNA is damaged. The protein kinases ataxia telangiectasia mutated (ATM) and Chk2, which phosphorylate and stabilize p53, are subsequently activated by this mechanism. P53 gathers (accumulated) in the nucleus and uses DNA binding to influence transcription. There are numerous additional variables that can activate p53. Anomalous growth signals have the ability to activate p53. The tumor suppressor p14 ARF, a protein that can bind the p53 inhibitor Mdm2 and prevent it from interacting with p53, is stimulated to express in response to these signals. Kinases involved in the control of Mdm2 can also trigger p53 in response to oxidative and metabolic stresses. A number of these kinases also serve as posttranscriptional modifiers, changing the structure and stability of the p53 protein by adding or removing moieties. Many secondary effects of P53 include suppression of neovascularization, induction of apoptosis, and control of the cell cycle. P53 has the ability to impede cell cycle progression by inducing the CDKI p21. A strong inhibitor of CDK, which is engaged in the Rb pathway, is p21. P53 contributes to apoptosis by upregulating the expression of cell surface markers like PIDD, Fas, and Killer/DR5. Proteins including NOXA, BAX, and p53AIP1, which impair mitochondrial function and accelerate cell death, are also expressed as a result of P53. P53 can stimulate the production of maspin and thrombospondin 1, two essential proteins that prevent neovascularization. Several substances are now undergoing testing due to their wide spectrum of effects that are essential for tumor suppression to give mutant p53 their actual functionality again. The protein Mdm2 generally controls P53 function. In addition to binding to p53, this protein has the ability to ubiquitinate, marking it for proteasomal breakdown. P53 causes an upregulation of Mdm2, which inhibits negative feedback. ATM and Chk2 have the ability to phosphorylate Mdm2 and so block its impact on p53. The antisense RNA Wrap53 also regulates P53 after transcription. In the presence of DNA damage, Wrap53 attaches itself to the p53 mRNA to stabilize it. Significantly lower amounts of p53 target synthesis are seen in Wrap53 knockdown models, indicating that Wrap53 is crucial for raising p53 levels (Farnebo et al., 2010).

There are several ways that malignancy might modify TP53 function. There can be no functional gene product from direct nonsense mutations. A nonfunctional protein that binds to a functional p53 and inactivates it can be produced by missense mutations. Moreover, mutations in the mdm2 regulatory pathway have been noted. Reduced function is also a result of mutations in the p53 downstream effectors. p53 function is essential for a cell to be able to cycle through the cell cycle properly or, if required, trigger apoptosis. Several TTAGGG DNA repeats, a 3' overhang, and a variety of related binding proteins make up telomeres. Among the many functions of telomeres is the preservation of chromosomal integrity and the promotion of DNA replication. In addition to providing a 5' template for priming DNA polymerase, the shape of telomeres prevents the DDR system from misinterpreting chromosomal ends as double-strand breaks, enabling precise chromosomal replication.

6.8. Telomere Biology

The dynamic length of telomeres suppresses tumor growth. Two enzymes, telomerase reverse transcriptase (TERT) and telomerase RNA component (TERC), are responsible for maintaining telomeres at the ends of each chromosome. TERT activity is correlated with telomere synthesis. Only hematological, epithelial, and activated lymphocytes and stem cells show significant TERT activity in adult humans. With every cell cycle in the absence of these enzymes, telomeres are continuously broken down. Eventually, a double-strand break occurs when exposed double-stranded DNA is detected by the cell. When the DDR system detects this, p53 is activated. Following this irreversible double-strand break, normal cells will either experience apoptosis or enter senescence. The specific senescence mechanism varies significantly between tissues and may involve activation of NK cells, AKT, or p16. Alternatively, when the telomeres have been damaged, cells may continue to proliferate slowly. This causes a phenomenon known as telomere crisis, which terminates in the development of severe genomic instability and cell death. Investigations into dysplastic tissues, like colonic adenomas, have revealed significant genomic instability, low TERT function, and telomere degradation. Rarely can cells pass through this slow proliferative phase without experiencing any additional limitations on their ability to proliferate. This leads to immortalization, as evidenced by cell lines from humans, yeast, and mice. Human cancer cells have the capacity to preserve some degree of telomere integrity and are uniformly immortalized. Most of these immortalized cells have partially recovered their TERT function. Although TERT reactivation is the main mechanism observed in cancer, 10–15% of cancers are believed to use an alternate telomere biosynthesis mechanism called alternative lengthening of telomeres (ALT) (Sohn et al., 2023).

The telomere (Figure 6.3) is reconstituted by homologous recombination-based exchange of telomeres throughout multiple cell division cycles. PML nuclear structures, extrachromosomal telomeric DNA, and extremely heterogeneous chromosomal length are characteristics of ALT-undergoing cells. Recombination precise mechanisms are not fully known. The telomerase length serves as an essential defense against neoplastic transformation and immortalization. Cancers can evade this system by reactivating TERC or by using the ALT pathway, which permits unrestricted replication. Four members make up the transmembrane receptor tyrosine kinases called epidermal growth factor receptor (EGFR) family: HER1, HER2, HER3, and HER4. Except for HER3, the molecular architectures of EGFRs consist of an intracellular domain that has tyrosine kinase (TK) activity, a short transmembrane domain, and an external ligand-binding domain. Different ligands, including TGF-alpha and epidermal growth factor (EGF), attach to the extracellular domain to start a signal transduction cascade that causes cell proliferation, anti-apoptotic signals, adhesion, migration, and differentiation, as well as the advancement of the cell cycle. Both heterodimerization with different HER protein types and homodimerization with EGFR are induced by ligand attachment to the EGFR extracellular domain. Although it is the preferred heterodimerization partner for other HER family members, HER2 does not bind to any known ligands.

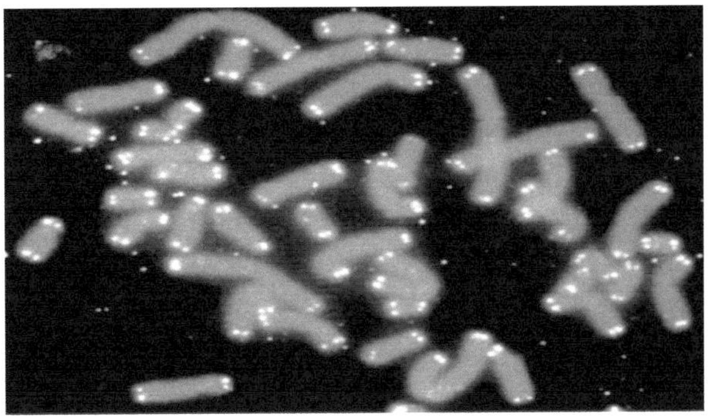

Figure 6.3. *Telomere.*

Source: https://upload.wikimedia.org/wikipedia/commons/4/4a/Telomere_caps.gif, Creative Commons License.

HER2 overexpression has been connected to a worse prognosis for gastric cancer, just like it does for breast cancer. The 5-year survival rates for HER2-positive and HER2-negative gastric cancer, respectively, were reported in Japan to be 11% and 50%, respectively. It was demonstrated that HER2 expression levels significantly correlated with overall survival and that HER2 was an independent prognostic marker in gastric cancer that had been removed. According to reports, intestinal gastric cancer has higher HER2/neu-positivity rates than diffuse gastric cancer or mixed kinds. In gastric cancer, HER2/neu amplification is generally linked to a poor prognosis. A monoclonal antibody called trastuzumab specifically targets the HER2 protein by attaching itself to the receptor extracellular domain. Patients with HER2-positive breast cancer, including primary and metastatic, had higher survival rates when treated with trastuzumab. Due to the success in treating breast cancer with the molecule, patients with HER2-positive malignancies such as gastric and GEJ adenocarcinomas are now being studied for the drug's potential antitumor effects. Trastuzumab therapy decreased the development of gastric cancer cell lines in preclinical investigations.

The most common method of MMR gene inactivation in cases of sporadic colorectal cancer is biallelic inactivation by methylation and transcriptional suppression of the MLH1 promoter region. MSI status can be determined by PCR-based DNA testing for MSI to determine instability at microsatellite sequences, or by immunohistochemistry to measure expression of DNA mismatch repair proteins. Finding out whether an MSI-positive tumor with loss of MLH1 expression is likely to be an inherited Lynch syndrome/HNPCC tumor or sporadic-type CRC depends on combining testing for BRAF V600E activating mutation and CpG island methylation status of the promoter region of the MLH1 gene. One interesting feature of MSI is its unique correlation with colon cancer behavior. It was demonstrated that MSI occurs in 17% of cases of colon cancer in individuals under 50 years of age (Chou et al., 2010). This MSI was linked to a decreased risk of tumor metastasis to nearby lymph nodes as well as distant organs, which resulted in an overall survival advantage regardless of the disease stage. MSI-H tumors had a better overall prognosis, were more likely to be in younger patients, poorly differentiated with mucin formation, and be less advanced than MSI-low level cancers. Apart from its prognostic function, MSI also has a predictive role. Chemotherapy was found to reduce advanced stage III colorectal tumors that had MSI-H. Further investigations revealed that patients receiving fluorouracil (5-FU) for stage II cancers with insufficient DNA mismatch repair and, thus, an MSI-positive status did not experience an increase in disease-free survival; on the contrary, treatment was linked to a decrease in overall survival. To be clear about the usefulness of these markers for treatment selection in ordinary patient care, larger trials are required. However, patients with stage II CRC who may benefit from chemotherapy should not use 5-FU alone in their treatment regimens.

6.9. Mutations and Response

In colorectal cancer (CRC), activating mutations of genes involved in the EGFR signaling pathways are the main cause of abnormal activation of these pathways, which occurs often. Since activating mutations in the EGFR gene are not a characteristic of CRC, tyrosine kinase inhibitors that target the EGFR, such as gefitinib and erlotinib, have not been demonstrated to have therapeutic efficacy in this disease.

About 40–45% of colorectal tumors include KRAS mutations, which are primarily located at exon 2, with rare mutations also occurring in codons 61 and 146. About 5–10% of all colorectal tumors have BRAF mutations, which are frequently observed in exon 15 with thymine (T) to adenine (A) transversion at nucleotide position 1796.

This mutation results in the replacement of valine for glutamate, or V600E. Significantly, the BRAF V600E mutation is present in 4–12% of microsatellite stable tumors that are capable of DNA mismatch repair and in 40–74% of sporadic MSI-H CRCs that are MLH1-deficient; however, it is not present in MLH1-deficient MSI-H CRCs that are associated with Lynch syndrome or HNPCC. About 20% of cases of colon cancer are found to have PI3K axis mutations. Mutations in genes can coexist in around 5% of cancers, demonstrating that mutations in the two EGFR signaling axes are not mutually exclusive. Many studies have been conducted on the function of EGFR gene mutations in the clinical management of colorectal cancer. Because KRAS mutations occur early in the development of cancer, they do not by themselves indicate a poor prognosis. Comparing BRAF mutations to wild-type BRAF tumors, however, indicates a significantly worse prognosis. It is not possible to inform if the mutations in the PI3K axis are predictive of CRC prognosis. The EGFR pathway is becoming a significant target for therapy. Anti-EGFR antibodies that target the receptor extracellular domain include cetuximab and panitumumab. They have been demonstrated to enhance survival and progression-free survival with metastatic colorectal cancer. Cetuximab treatment significantly increased overall survival in patients with wild-type KRAS tumors when compared to supportive care alone. There was no statistically significant distinction between individuals with mutant KRAS tumors treated with cetuximab and those who did not. Some studies found that while individuals with wild-type KRAS colorectal cancer benefited from cetuximab therapy, those with mutant KRAS colorectal tumors did not. Because constitutive activation of KRAS leads to release from EGFR and because activated KRAS is downstream of the latter, KRAS mutations make these agents ineffective. These trials showed that tumors with KRAS mutation in codons 12, 13, or 61 did not benefit from treatment with cetuximab or panitumumab (Er et al., 2014). In wild-type CRC, anti-EGFR therapy has a response rate of up to 40%. The other 60% of wild-type tumors do not react to anti-EGFR therapy, most likely as a result of gene/protein changes in the EGFR or other signaling pathways.

6.10. Drugs and the Mutational Status

Many drugs that may inhibit downstream signaling pathways are being investigated for CRC with an active mutant KRAS. It is still uncertain how BRAF mutational tests will predict CRC. Although BRAF-activating mutations should function similarly to KRAS in terms of EGFR antibody therapy response, it is challenging to evaluate this role due to the poor prognosis that a BRAF mutation confers and the relatively small percentage of cases with BRAF mutations in clinical trials. Larger clinical trials are required to ascertain if colorectal cancer will respond to BRAF inhibitors in a manner akin to that currently observed in melanoma, although these drugs have been evaluated in preliminary investigations. By using fast feedback activation of EGFR, which reduces the benefit of vemurafenib, it has recently been shown that colon cancer cells, as opposed to melanoma cells, are insensitive to the BRAF inhibitor vemurafenib. Therefore, to affect clinical responses in BRAF-mutant CRC, a combined strategy focusing on EGFR and BRAF may be required. Preclinical evidence indicates that cancer cells become resistant to cetuximab when they harbor a PIK3CA/PTEN mutation, which results in activation of the PI3K pathway. Preclinical research demonstrates that PIK3CA mutations decouple cell proliferation signaling from the KRAS pathway, which results in the ineffectiveness of inhibitors that target the MAPK axis. PIK3CA mutation is related to poor response to cetuximab, contrary to the initial small studies that suggested conflicting roles of PIK3CA mutation in response to EGFR antibodies. Preclinical models suggest that PI3K axis suppression might be necessary in these tumors to control the cancer. It has been demonstrated that blocking the PI3K pathway in cancer cells with activating PI3KCA mutations inhibits cell proliferation and triggers apoptosis. BRAF, NRAS, and PIK3CA exon mutations are significantly linked to a low response rate to cetuximab targeted therapy. Simultaneous inhibition with MEK and AKT/PI3K inhibitors is necessary to regulate cell proliferation when mutations exist in both EGFR pathway axes (McCubrey et al., 2012). Since activating EGFR mutations in CRC do not confer susceptibility to tyrosine kinase inhibitors or cetuximab therapy, EGFR mutational testing is not recommended for CRC. It has been noted that cetuximab has a response in colorectal cancer patients whose tumors do not express the epidermal growth factor receptor, indicating that EGFR IHC is not necessary for patient selection or exclusion from cetuximab therapy. The KRAS mutational status is the main criterion used to identify CRC patients with metastatic disease who are candidates for targeted therapy using anti-EGFR antibodies. The way that anti-EGFR targeted therapy works may depend on the mutational status of BRAF, NRAS, PI3KCA, and other genes downstream of EGFR.

Usage of cetuximab among patients with chemotherapy-refractory colon cancer with the KRAS G13D mutation may be related to prolonged overall and progression-free survival, but this is still questionable. This is in contrast to other activating variants in KRAS. Since KRAS mutations occur early in the genesis of colorectal carcinogenesis, most clinical trials tested the primary tumor site when selecting tissue for DNA mutational analysis. Published studies revealed a strong correlation between the KRAS mutation status in primary vs. metastatic colon cancer lesions, with a high average concordance of 93%. It is reasonable to evaluate tumor tissue from either the main site or from metastatic lesions. It is recommended that pathologists choose a block of formalin-fixed, paraffin-embedded (FFPE) tissue that has the highest percentage of viable tumors and the largest feasible tumor area. Depending on the assay being used, different laboratories may have varying requirements. Technical methods for mutational testing differ greatly between labs and adhere to validation and interpretation guidelines, especially for tests produced in the lab. Sanger sequencing, allele-specific PCR, pyrosequencing, fluorescent bead detection assay, melt curve analysis, MassARRAY MALDI-TOF mass spectrometry, and more recent next-generation deep sequencing techniques are examples of these techniques. By combining macro- or micro-dissected tissue from various tissue levels, an adequate amount of DNA can be produced. A biopsy may be better than the resection material if the resection was carried out following neoadjuvant therapy, and the tissue would not be suitable for genetic testing if there were only a few remaining tumor cells. When patients are candidates for targeted anti-EGFR antibody therapy, KRAS mutational screening of CRC tumor tissues is advised.

Published research suggests that additional mutational testing of other EGFR pathway genes may be useful to better select patients for targeted therapy with improved results, however, there is still no agreement regarding which genes should be investigated. Large labs are testing all colorectal adenocarcinomas for microsatellite instability, BRAF V600E mutations, and KRAS codon 12–13 alterations. This allows for patient selection for both targeted therapy and conventional therapy. Barrett's metaplasia (BM) is a disorder caused by chronic gastroesophageal reflux disease (GERD) in which the squamous lining (esophagus) is replaced with specialized columnar epithelium containing goblet cells. A higher risk of esophageal adenocarcinoma (EAC) is linked to BM (Lindkvist et al., 2014). Since the 1970s, the prevalence of EAC has increased in Western Europe and the United States. Although the majority of EAC cases are diagnosed at a late stage and have a wrong prognosis, survival rates have been steadily rising over time. Patients with BM are part of monitoring programs, in which biopsy and esophageal endoscopy are done at predetermined intervals, mostly based on the level of dysplasia in the biopsy tissue. Effective prevention and treatment efforts require an understanding of the molecular alterations that take place as normal squamous epithelium progresses to BM and ultimately to EAC. Bile and acid are involved in both the neoplastic and metaplastic processes. Acid reflux can stimulate the NADPH oxidase NOX5-S and produce more reactive oxygen species, which can then upregulate p16 expression, methylate the p16 promoter, and promote cell division. It has been demonstrated that in cultured human cell lines, acidic pH enhances the expression of COX-2 in the squamous epithelium and induces topoisomerase-II (TOP2)-mediated DNA damage and p53 protein overexpression.

Acid suppression treatment appears to not affect oxidative DNA damage, apoptosis, the expression of COX-2, c-myc, p53, O6-methylguanine methyltransferase (MGMT), or aberrant DNA methylation, but it does lower heartburn, inflammation, and proliferative activity in BM. Bile acids, particularly Deoxycholic acid (DCA), induce mutations in the human p53 gene and cause chromosome damage via reactive oxygen species (ROS), both at neutral and acidic pH levels. However, the effects of acidic pH are high. Acid suppression therapy may not completely eradicate DNA damage or the carcinogenic potential of redox fluoride since bile acids can cause damage to DNA even at neutral pH levels. Bile acids also cause NF-kappaB to be activated in BM. In BM epithelial cells, DCA causes genotoxicity and activates the NF-kappaB pathway at the same time, preventing apoptosis in cells that have sustained DNA damage.

6.11. Gene Expression and Response

An essential function of the caudal-related homeobox genes CDX1 and CDX2 is intestinal epithelial differentiation. CDX1 and CDX2 mRNA are expressed in gastric intestinal metaplasia. Mouse oesophageal keratinocytes exhibit transcription of the CDX2 gene when exposed to an acidic pH. In a rat model, cholic, and deoxycholic acids induce the synthesis of intestinal-type mucin and CDX2 protein in oesophageal keratinocytes via activating the CDX2 promoter via NF-kappaB. Acid and deoxycholate stimulate NF-kappaB activity in cultured human EAC cell lines, which in turn causes CDX2 production. CDX2 then promotes intestinal metaplasia and the expression of guanylyl cyclase C (GC-C), an intestinal-specific tumor suppressor. While CDX2 protein is exclusively found in BM in human biopsy tissue, CDX2 mRNA is present in both BM and esophagitis epithelium. The expression of CDX1 mRNA is limited to BM epithelium. The methylation state of the CDX1 promoter is assumed to be the cause of the specific expression of CDX1 mRNA in only BM and not in the squamous or gastric epithelium (Poehlmann et al., 2012). The expression of CDX1 mRNA can be increased *in vitro* by conjugated bile salts, TNFalpha, and IL-1beta through NF-kappaB signaling, but only *in situ*ations where the CDX1 promoter is unmethylated or partially methylated. Recently, there has been a proposal that factors produced by fibroblasts can cause the neighboring squamous epithelium to exhibit a columnar phenotype. Heparin-binding EGF-like growth factor (HB-EGF) is upregulated in human bone marrow cells exposed to acidic media. The biopsy samples obtained from individuals suffering from reflux esophagitis exhibit a prominent manifestation of HB-EGF in the fibroblasts beneath the injured epithelium. Moreover, HB-EGF stimulates HET1A human squamous epithelial cells *in vitro*, upregulating villin and cytokeratin in addition to increasing

CDX2 expression in a dose-dependent way. It has been suggested that CDX2 may function as a marker of BM *in situ*ations where intestinal metaplasia is absent from the biopsy because CDX2 expression has been found in columnar cells with intestinal metaplasia and those that do not exhibit it in many studies of esophageal biopsies. Researchers hypothesized that CDX2 expression in cardiac-type mucosa may serve as an indicator for the presence of intestinal metaplasia without goblet cells by predicting the presence of undetected intestinal metaplasia in columnar lined esophagus.

It was discovered that BM expressed cyclin D1, and that patients taking antacids, proton pump inhibitors (PPI), and H2-blockers had less cyclin D1 expression. PPIs lowered Cyclin D1 levels, which was then followed by H2-blockers and antacids, which had the least impact. Aggressive tumors, early cancer initiation, and elevated Cyclin D1 expression are linked to the adenine 870 polymorphism in Cyclin D1. Via ligand-dependent transactivation of the epidermal growth factor receptor (EGFR), deoxycholic acid induces CDX2. *In vitro*, DCA can upregulate EGFR mRNA at neutral pH, acidic pH, or pH alone. In the case of neutral pH DCA, NF-kappaB was required. By using semiquantitative IHC, it was discovered that, in comparison to BM, EGFR was overexpressed in 80% of EAC and 35% of BM with high-grade dysplasia (HGD). EGFR overexpression was associated with both chromosomal aneuploidy and EGFR locus amplification. The Raf/MEK/ERK (MAPK) kinase pathway, which may be triggered early in the development of Barrett's adenocarcinoma, partially mediates EGFR signaling. About 32% of all Barrett's adenocarcinomas and a percentage of lesions with high-grade dysplasia had RAS or BRAF mutations. c-erbB2 was discovered to be amplified in dysplastic BM and a significant number of EAC, both by IHC and FISH. Immunostaining and amplification revealed significant variation in EAC and dysplastic foci. In almost half of the cases of EAC and BM with HGD, some researchers discovered that polysomy 17 without Her-2/neu gene amplification was linked to neither weak nor normal immunostaining nor normal or moderately enhanced mRNA expression. In cases of BM with low-grade dysplasia (LGD), there was no locus-specific Her-2/neu amplification; however, polysomy 17 was observed, indicating that chromosome 17 polysomy without Her-2/neu gene amplification precedes Her-2/neu gene amplification in HGD and EAC (Younes, 2013). The FISH measurement of the HER-2/neu oncogene amplification is correlated with a reduced patient survival rate and independently predicts an inconclusive prognosis for individuals with EAC. Patients treated with trastuzumab and conventional chemotherapy in patients with positive Her2/neu exhibited a significant survival benefit, which included stomach and gastroesophageal junction adenocarcinomas.

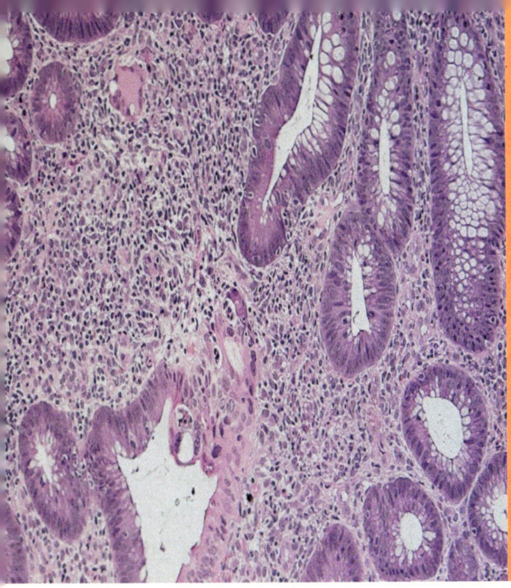

Chapter 7

DRUG THERAPY FOR GI DISEASES

Contents

7.1. Introduction

A frequent condition known as gastro-oesophageal reflux disease (GORD) is brought on by the retrograde passage of stomach contents through a gastro-oesophageal junction (incompetent) (Tack and Pandolfino, 2018). It includes a broad spectrum of symptoms, ranging from severe esophagitis to endoscopy-negative disease, or symptoms without lesions at endoscopy. The common symptom, heartburn, along with regurgitation affects 10–20% of adults. Only 1–4% of cases, however, have moderate to severe symptoms. A large number of patients who experience sporadic heartburn and/or regurgitation choose to self-treat using over-the-counter medications like antacids and, more recently, H2-receptor antagonists rather than seeking medical attention. Esophagitis, on the other hand, is less common, perhaps affecting 2% of the general population and impacting no more than 30–50% of patients who are sent to an endoscopic unit due to symptoms indicative of GORD. The majority of individuals who have mucosal breaks during endoscopy have non-circumferential lesions, or mild to moderate esophagitis. Particularly in young people, severe esophagitis or deep ulcers are rare. A serious consequence of GORD is intestinal metaplasia of the distal esophageal mucosa, yet there are additional elements involved in its etiology as well. While systematic biopsies from the cardia often reveal metaplasia, fewer than 10% of patients undergoing endoscopy for reflux symptoms have Barrett's esophagus, or columnar-lined esophagitis (3 cm or more). Barrett's esophagus is a premalignant disorder that increases the chance of esophageal adenocarcinoma by 30 to 40 times, although it is often asymptomatic and not always linked to the macroscopic alterations of esophagitis. Malignant development follows a path that starts with metaplasia, progresses to dysplasia, and ends with carcinoma.

7.2. The Biology of Gastro-Oesophageal Reflux Disease

The therapy of GORD has advanced significantly over the past 10 years, due to the discovery of proton pump inhibitors (PPIs). The disease, which is typically a chronic relapsing disorder, cannot be cured by any of the medications now prescribed for anti-reflux therapy. GORD can significantly lower a patient's quality of life, even in the absence of esophagitis lesions. Most of the reflux episodes occur during the temporary relaxations of the lower esophageal sphincter (TLOSRs) when the pressure within the LOS (lower esophageal sphincter) is at rest. Both the total number of TLOSRs and the percentage of relaxations linked to acid reflux appear to be higher in GORD patients than in healthy individuals with physiologically significant levels of acid reflux. No prokinetic medication now in use can alter the underlying aberrant motor pattern associated with GORD. TLOSRs are produced by the distension of mechanical receptors found in the proximal stomach wall, particularly in the sub cardiac region. This distension initiates a vagovagal response (reflux). Many drugs can reduce the rate of TLOSRs brought on by a meal or stomach distension with air in pharmacological studies done on humans or animals. Although the presence of non-specific adverse effects, such as the development of drowsiness about the central action of morphinomimetic compounds, hinders the use of these compounds in clinical practice, they offer promise for more reasonable pharmacological therapy in the future. The important impact of acid and pepsin action on the esophageal mucosa, in addition to aberrant motility, has been fully validated by the effect of acid suppression provided by PPIs in GORD. The etiology of reflux esophagitis may also involve non-acid components of the gastric refluxate. Therefore, bile acids can increase the harmful effects of pepsin and acid, leading to more severe damage to the mucosa. However, acidic, and non-acidic substances work at low pH values rather than at alkaline pH values. For this reason, pH monitoring is not a suitable method for studying enterogastro-esophageal reflux (Hanna et al., 2014). Therefore, the decrease in gastric capacity brought about by PPI medication is likely advantageous for both acid and non-acid reflux.

7.3. Helicobacter pylori

Helicobacter pylori has been shown to play a crucial role in the pathology of peptic ulcer disease, although this is not the case with GORD. The bacteria do not appear to be a factor in the motility problems, such as raising the rate of TLOSRs or changing the timing of stomach emptying, which appears to be delayed in roughly 40% of GORD patients. Eliminating the *Helicobacter pylori* infection may necessitate a higher PPI dosage in patients suffering from reflux esophagitis to regulate acid output. Formulations known as antacids are primarily made to counteract stomach acid. The common ways to administer antacids are in the form of tablets, while other formulations come in the form of gels. The antacid component in liquid formulations can either be insoluble and present as a fine solid such as aluminum hydroxide or soluble in water such as sodium bicarbonate. Tablets are thought to be less successful than liquid solutions in reducing stomach acidity. Due to their quick gastric emptying, antacids taken while fasting only have a short, temporary effect on stomach pH. They lessen acidity for about 30 minutes. The stomach pH remains over 2.0 for three hours when antacids (30 ml) are administered one and three hours after the meal. Even when taken before bedtime, antacids are unable to reduce the nocturnal gastric acidity, which often peaks after midnight. Certain antacids, particularly those that contain aluminum, cause the stomach to take longer to empty both liquids and solids. This inhibition could be viewed as a positive attribute since it is thought that the length of the neutralizing effect of liquid antacids is limited by how quickly they are emptied from the stomach. It is better to increase the frequency of delivery rather than the dose of antacid drug when a schedule proves to be ineffective. In clinical practice, using a suitable antisecretory treatment (PPIs) makes controlling acidity easier. Antacids may lessen gastric juice peptic activity.

More efficient in its ability to absorb bile salts is aluminum hydroxide. The chemical structure of the bile salt and conjugation have an impact on the binding affinity of the bile salts for antacids. Several prokinetic drugs have been tried in the past to treat GORD (Quigley, 2017). One cholinergic drug that has been proven to be useful in treating esophagitis in both adults and children is bethanechol. It also causes many adverse effects and increases the secretion of gastric acid. Similarly, metoclopramide, a 5HT3-antagonist, sometimes causes side effects like bowel disturbance, dizziness, and even severe extrapyramidal manifestations, even at relatively high doses that are beneficial in treating reflux symptoms. The dopamine antagonist domperidone, which is related to butyrophenones, exhibits pharmacodynamic effects on stomach and esophageal motility that are almost identical to those of metoclopramide. Domperidone rarely produces extrapyramidal effects and does not penetrate the blood-brain barrier, however, it can cause hyperprolactinemia symptoms like galactorrhea or amenorrhea. In GORD, outcomes comparable to those of metoclopramide would be anticipated, with domperidone exhibiting good tolerability. Metoclopramide and domperidone have essentially been abandoned as treatments for gastrointestinal motility disorders, however, they are still used for dyspepsia and other associated diseases.

7.4. Cisapride

Cisapride has prokinetic properties without having an antidopaminergic impact. It is an agonist of 5-HT4 receptors and causes the gut myenteric plexus to produce acetylcholine. Cisapride accelerates stomach emptying, raises LOS pressure, particularly in reflux patients with low baseline tone, and amplifies esophageal body contractions. Cisapride, however, has no effect on the rate of TLOSRs. Cisapride has a slight effect on gastric acid secretion, despite its indirect cholinomimetic effects. In asymptomatic volunteers, cisapride increases salivary secretion. This impact might help patients with GORD by promoting esophageal clearance.

Cisapride is effective for treating both adults and children. For the temporary alleviation of esophagitis symptoms and healing, cisapride (10 mg four times a day) works better than a placebo and is on par with H2-receptor antagonists. Cisapride lowers the 6- and 12-month relapse incidence of esophagitis (Blum et al., 1993). However, the majority of individuals with mild to severe esophagitis are not able to benefit from the therapy. The most common side effects of cisapride include headache, mild diarrhea, and abdominal pain, all of which are generally easily tolerated. However, there have been new reports of unusual but fatal cardiac problems, such as torsades de pointes. This side effect could significantly lessen the effectiveness of cisapride in the treatment of GORD. The doctor should also be aware of the interactions that exist between cisapride and many other drugs, including ketoconazole and spiramycin, for which it is strictly prohibited to take both at the same time. Due to potentially fatal cardiac side effects, the production license for cisapride has recently been revoked in several European and American countries. Short-term studies have looked into the use of metoclopramide and cimetidine in combination therapy. The clinical and endoscopic outcomes attained by mixing this prokinetic substance with cimetidine are often not better than those attained with cimetidine alone. H2-receptor antagonists have also been used in combination with the modern prokinetic drug cisapride. A trend toward improvement was observed when ranitidine was paired with cisapride. In comparison to H2-receptor antagonist monotherapy, further controlled trials showing cisapride added to either cimetidine or ranitidine produced noticeably higher healing rates. When cisapride – 10 mg three times daily was added to ranitidine – 150 mg twice daily in maintenance therapy, the relapse rate at 12 months was considerably lower than when ranitidine was used alone. Adding cisapride to omeprazole produced better results than combination therapy with ranitidine, although the relapse rate found with ranitidine plus cisapride was not statistically different from that observed with omeprazole alone. However, omeprazole monotherapy by itself appears to be more economical for long-term heartburn relief than combined therapy with H2-receptor antagonists (Boparai et al., 2008).

7.5. Drug Combinations

There are not many applications for prokinetic and antisecretory drug combinations. However, in certain patients, such as those whose primary complaint is regurgitation, this method might be useful. There is currently a chewable version of cimetidine available. This new formulation showed a very rapid action; the average time for some improvement was less than 20 minutes, and the medium time for complete pain alleviation was less than 45 minutes. It was also discovered that a chewable tablet with cimetidine and alginic acid was useful in reducing GORD symptoms. For quicker symptom alleviation, effervescent tablets might potentially be an effective treatment option. An effervescent version of ranitidine or cimetidine has been made accessible in recent years. These effervescent preparations have the benefit of rapidly reducing intragastric acidity by combining the immediate action of a pH buffer with the longer-lasting systemic effect of an H2-receptor blockage.

7.6. Other Molecules

Recently, famotidine is being used in clinical settings. It was meant to dissolve quickly on the tongue and be ingested without water. Compliance should rise as a result of this simplicity of administration, particularly in patients who have trouble swallowing. Since tablets have been demonstrated to lodge in the esophagus in at least 20% of the patients, the famotidine wafer, together with the cimetidine and ranitidine effervescent formulations, would also help to avoid the issues associated with poor esophageal transit of conventional forms. While lansoprazole, pantoprazole, and rabeprazole have been introduced more recently, omeprazole was the first PPI widely tested for the treatment of reflux esophagitis. The final enzyme in the production of gastric acid, gastric H+/K+-ATPase, interacts with all of these substituted benzimidazoles. This inhibition of the proton pump offers a better way to regulate the release of acid. Lipophilic weak bases called substituted benzimidazoles are absorbed from the small intestine and go through the bloodstream to the gastric parietal cells. Since PPIs do not alter at physiological pH, they can pass through cell membranes. But, when PPIs are exposed to a pH lower than 2, they stop being lipophilic and get trapped and concentrated in the acidic milieu of the canaliculus of the actively secreting gastric parietal cell. PPIs do not directly inhibit H+/K+-ATPase; rather, as the pH drops, the protonated versions of the drugs change into the active form, cationic sulfenamide (Sachs, 1997). The enzyme is made inactive by the sulfenamide reaction with cysteines on the proton pump extracellular surface. *In vivo*, this covalent interaction is irreversible; the synthesis of fresh H+/K+-ATPase protein is the only way that acid secretion can resume. Because the proton pump half-life in humans can be around 18 hours, this accounts for the prolonged antisecretory effect of PPIs.

All PPIs that are currently on the market have somewhat comparable pharmacokinetics, showing a high percentage of protein binding and a short half-life of roughly one hour. Only pantoprazole and rabeprazole exhibit dose-linearity, whereas lansoprazole and pantoprazole seem to have a higher bioavailability. Food does not seem to alter the bioavailability of PPIs, although taking antacids at the same time as taking PPIs causes omeprazole and lansoprazole to absorb more slowly. The cytochrome P450 system metabolizes pantoprazole, lansoprazole, and omeprazole, with the inactive metabolites being eliminated in the urine. However, in cases of renal or hepatic failure, dosage modifications are typically not required. The interaction of omeprazole and lansoprazole with the cytochrome P450 system should be considered when drugs such as diazepam are administered concurrently, even if it has minimal therapeutic significance. There do not seem to be any drug-to-drug interactions with the PPIs, pantoprazole, and rabeprazole. Many investigations have demonstrated that PPIs reduce acid secretion. But unlike with H2-receptor antagonists, there is often a nocturnal breakthrough, meaning that the stomach pH stays below pH 4.35 during this time. It was discovered that adding ranitidine to omeprazole was a very effective way to combat this nocturnal acid breakthrough issue. It is better to try adding an H2-receptor antagonist to Barrett's esophagitis patients who do not respond well to PPI treatment, even though the importance of this phenomenon in GORD is still uncertain. The situation of duodenal ulcers is complex. Although increased acid secretion is a major contributing component, the etiology has been linked to other factors as well, such as gender, genetic susceptibility, alcohol, and drug use, smoking, and, most recently, *H. pylori* infection. A series of synergistic pathogenetic processes make up the pathophysiology of duodenal ulcers. The majority of individuals with duodenal ulcers have antral-predominant active chronic gastritis and are colonized by *H. pylori* strains that are typically virulent. When paired with accelerated stomach emptying, antral *H. pylori* infection reduces the inhibitory feedback control of acid secretion, increasing the duodenal acid load. Active duodenitis arises when *H. pylori* colonizes these duodenal foci of gastric metaplasia.

7.7. Ulcers

Ulcers may occasionally form in conjunction with other irritating elements such as NSAIDs if duodenitis worsens to the point where the inflamed mucosa is unable to preserve its structural integrity (Sergi, 2020). The amount of gastric acid produced is correlated with the degree of gastric metaplasia. Treatments intended to lower acidity are ineffective against duodenitis, and the mucosa of the duodenum that heals is not histologically normal. Gastritis does not alter stomach metaplasia. The elimination of *H. pylori* results in the remission of duodenal inflammation, just like in chronic gastritis. The duodenal ulcer heals, the mucosal defense returns, and there is no more ulcer recurrence when there is no *H. pylori* infection. Following the infection resolution, acid secretion only partially returns to normal, which likely explains the frequently observed incomplete resolution of stomach metaplasia. Patients who have stomach ulcers typically exhibit a distinct gastritis pattern. Unlike duodenal ulcers, which are limited to the antrum, gastritis typically affects the corpus mucosa, causing different degrees of atrophy. This reduces the corpus mucosal capacity to secrete acid. The corpus of the stomach is unable to react to the gastrin stimulus, even if inflammation of the antrum in these patients causes increased gastrin secretion. Since most people with stomach ulcers have relatively low acid flow, excess acid is not the etiology of proximal gastric ulcers. It is likely that the acid-secreting mucosal resistance to local acid generation, even at low levels, is compromised by the inflammation caused by *H. pylori*. After *H. pylori* is eliminated, acid output sometimes returns to normal. Gastritis caused by *H. pylori* is becoming less common in Western countries. Currently, the majority of gastric ulcers are brought on by drugs, mostly aspirin and other non-steroidal anti-inflammatory drugs (NSAIDs). A significant proportion of *H. pylori*-negative stomach ulcers are caused by the ingestion of these drugs. Reactive gastritis or NSAID use is linked to 26–45% of foveolar hyperplasia, edema, splaying of muscle fibers in the lamina propria, vasodilatation, congestion, and lack of inflammatory cells. It is unknown why some people experience reactive gastritis after taking NSAIDs, but it is not linked to *H. pylori*. The best way to determine the impact of *H. pylori* on NSAID-induced gastroduodenal mucosal injury is to assess the ulcer recurrence rate following *H. pylori* removal and subsequent NSAID reuse. More suitable clinical trials in patients at risk for ulcers and related consequences are necessary to determine whether the pathophysiologic interaction between *H. pylori* and NSAIDs is clinically effective.

7.8. Histamine

When histamine from mast cells and enterochromaffin-like (ECL) cells occupy H2-receptors, adenylate cyclase is activated, raising intracellular concentrations of cyclic AMP. The parietal cell proton pump is activated by these elevated cyclic AMP levels, secreting hydrogen ions against a concentration gradient in return for potassium ions. By competitively and specifically blocking histamine binding to the receptor, H2RAs lower intracellular cyclic AMP concentrations and the acid production of parietal cells. H2RAs only partially suppress the stimulation of gastrin, acetylcholine, or histamine-induced acid secretion; this is likely due to a decrease in the secretion that happens when these stimuli are given simultaneously. The secretory membrane of the parietal cell is the only place where the proton pump, also known as the H+, K+-ATPase, is present. The proton pump is responsible for the parietal cell release of hydrochloric acid. Regardless of the kind or direction of the stimulus, the H+ and K+-ATPase translocate to the secretory canaliculus of the parietal cell plasma membrane during activation of the parietal cell. Since the extracellular portion of the pump is exposed to potassium ions, the parietal cells can secrete acid due to an increase in the membrane permeability to potassium. PPIs stop H+, K+-ATPase from working. PPIs have a stronger antisecretory action than H2RA and regulate gastric acid output in a dose-dependent manner. Meta-analyses have demonstrated a strong relationship between ulcer healing and a decrease in intragastric acidity (Tunis et al., 1997). It seems that suppressing nighttime acidity is crucial for the repair of duodenal ulcers. Until recently, ulcers were treated with an acid suppression drug for a relatively short period of time to heal the ulcer, then for a longer period of time to avoid relapses. Recurrences of ulcers during maintenance therapy are frequently painless and may heal on their own with sustained therapy.

Eliminating *H. pylori* is advised for patients who test positive for the infection in order to avoid ulcer relapses and avoid costly maintenance therapy. Some patients, however, do not respond well to *H. pylori* treatment; others relapse after *H. pylori* is removed; still, others have co-morbid conditions that raise the risk of complications or recurrences; still, others are unwilling to finish an anti – *H. pylori* treatment regimen and require maintenance therapy. Duodenal ulcers that are *H. pylori*-negative are uncommon and should not be mistaken for false negatives. Inadequate mucosal biopsies or the patient's current use of drugs that suppress *H. pylori*, including PPIs or bismuth, can result in false-negative test results. False-negative test results can cause some *H. pylori* negative ulcers, but idiopathic causes, acid hypersecretion, and the surreptitious use of over-the-counter aspirin and NSAIDs are nonetheless significant contributors to ulcerogenesis. *H. pylori*-negative ulcers are uncommon and are distinguished by high serum gastrin, high acid-secretory capacity, and quick stomach emptying after all other variables have been ruled out. Acid suppressant drugs for ulcer healing and maintenance are recommended in these uncommon situations. Peptic ulcer therapy was previously limited to short-term acid suppression medication for healing and long-term maintenance therapy to avoid ulcer recurrence. *H. pylori* is found in more than 90% of patients with peptic ulcers, and evidence suggests that effective eradication therapy reduces the risk of ulcer-related complications and recurrence of ulcers. The treatment choices for peptic ulcer disease have undergone a significant shift due to these observations since antibiotic therapy has replaced acid suppression therapy. For patients with peptic ulcers linked to *H. pylori*, all current guidelines advise eliminating the infection. Regardless of whether the ulcer is active or in remission, treatment is necessary for all *H. pylori*-positive ulcers.

7.9. Intention-to-Treat Analysis

Intention-to-treat analysis (ITT) shows that no combination of drugs can completely remove *H. pylori* infection in over 85% of patients (Graham et al., 2008). Primary antibiotic resistance and patient compliance are the two most significant variables affecting the therapy's effectiveness. Treatment modalities are often categorized based on the quantity of drugs employed. PPI, or ranitidine bismuth citrate (RBC)-based triple treatments, are the best of these regimens; they typically yield 85–95% eradication rates. Because of the unacceptable low efficiency of the existing medications and the frequent formation of secondary bacterial resistance in those who are unable to eliminate the microorganism, monotherapy should never be utilized to eradicate *H. pylori*. With eradication rates of approximately 50%, clarithromycin is now the most effective antibiotic against *H. pylori* both *in vitro* and *in vivo*. However, two out of every three failures are caused by clarithromycin resistance. Using a PPI or H2RA in conjunction with one antibiotic, originally amoxicillin, but more recently clarithromycin, is known as dual therapy. Dual therapy produces unreliable results, typically less than 70%, and more successful regimens have since replaced it. A further dual therapy involves 14 days of clarithromycin and ranitidine bismuth citrate (RBC) administration. RBC is a ranitidine salt that has a high degree of water solubility. The bismuth and citrate combine to create a complex citrato-bismuth anion, with ranitidine serving as the cation. The antipepsin and anti-*H.pylori* impact of RBC is thought to be primarily related to its increased solubility, particularly at lower pH levels. Further, RBC plus clarithromycin 500 mg twice daily for 14 days is the most effective dosage schedule, with reported ITT eradication rates ranging from 76% to 96%. Two weeks of high-dose clarithromycin is an effective treatment, but it is costly and has a lot of side effects, which make compliance difficult.

7.10. Therapy

For many years, the standard treatment was bismuth-based triple therapy, which included a bismuth component, metronidazole, and tetracycline (or amoxicillin). With this regimen, eradication rates above 90% can be attained in just 14 days. The normal doses for metronidazole are 200–500 mg three times a day, tetracycline – 500 mg four times a day, and bismuth, four times a day. With a mean fall in efficacy from 97% to 44%, patients with metronidazole-resistant strains showed significantly lower eradication rates than patients with metronidazole-sensitive strains after receiving bismuth-tetracycline-metronidazole treatment for one or two weeks. It is safe and reasonably inexpensive to utilize empirical bismuth-based triple treatment for seven days where metronidazole resistance is known to be rare. Although improved eradication rates can be achieved using other regimens without imidazoles or by adding acid suppression to bismuth-based triple therapies, the course should be extended for 14 days where metronidazole resistance is highly prevalent. It is interesting to note that the *H. pylori* eradication rates rose from 52% to 84% in metronidazole-sensitive strains and from 39% to 64% in metronidazole-resistant strains when the dose of metronidazole in bismuth-based triple therapy was increased from 375 mg to 750 mg per day (Periti et al., 1999). Although the rate of side effects from bismuth-based triple therapy can range from 7% to 72%, only 3–3.5% of patients are forced to stop the therapy due to these adverse effects. Triple therapy based on bismuth has become less common because of its negative effects and complicated dosage schedule of four times each day. Triple therapy based on bismuth has the potential to be beneficial in resource-constrained places, but the high level of metronidazole resistance in these locations often results in subpar outcomes.

7.11. Addressing Challenges

An alternative is ranitidine-bismuth citrate (RBC), which combines bismuth antibacterial and cytoprotective qualities with ranitidine acid-suppressive capabilities. When combined with two antibiotics, clarithromycin – 250 mg daily and tetracycline – 500 mg twice daily, or amoxicillin 1 g twice daily for a maximum of seven days, RBC has been shown to be effective in eliminating *H. pylori*. With the 7-day regimens, the observed ITT eradication rates varied from 71% to 100%. The sensitivity to metronidazole does not seem to have a substantial impact on the *H. pylori* eradication rates for RBC and metronidazole with clarithromycin or tetracycline. For seven days, RBC- based triple therapy, clarithromycin plus either metronidazole or tetracycline, is a simple, efficient, and good treatment plan for *H. pylori* infection. Although the effectiveness of this regimen in cases of clarithromycin resistance has not been thoroughly investigated, available evidence indicates that four out of five strains of clarithromycin-resistant bacteria are eliminated when RBC-clarithromycin is combined with another antibiotic. One week of PPI-based triple therapy and one week of RBC-based triple therapy were equally effective. PPI-based triple treatment is currently the most used type, administered for seven days. PPI triple therapy mixes a PPI with any two of the three antibiotics, i.e., amoxicillin, clarithromycin, and nitroimidazole such as metronidazole or tinidazole. Omeprazole is the PPI that has been studied the most, but other PPIs appear to work just as well. Initially, a once-daily standard-dosage PPI was employed; however, randomized studies have shown that twice-daily doses, or a double-standard dose, are preferable. 30 mg twice a day of lansoprazole was found to be more effective than 15 mg twice a day when used in conjunction with clarithromycin and amoxicillin. When pantoprazole was taken twice daily in addition to the same antibiotics, it proved to be more effective than 40 mg once a day. Though the precise mechanisms are unclear, it is evident that adding an antisecretory drug increases the rates of *H. pylori* eradication.

Compared to patients with metronidazole-sensitive strains, patients with metronidazole-resistant strains tend to have lower eradication rates. Some investigations found a statistically significant drop in efficacy between sensitive and metronidazole-resistant bacteria. PPIs reduce side effects and dyspeptic symptoms in bismuth-based triple treatment. Despite being effective, quadruple therapy is primarily utilized as a second-line treatment following earlier unsuccessful therapies due to the intricacy of the regimen and a high number of tablets required. Until *H. pylori* is completely eradicated, second- or even third-line medications should be used if the first therapy is ineffective. Nevertheless, with the effectiveness of PPI triple, RBC triple, and quadruple therapy, there is a significant range in efficacy between treatment trials, with 95% confidence intervals falling between 80 and 100%. Up to 20% of patients in ordinary daily practice will not be able to eradicate *H. pylori* due to non-compliance, bacterial resistance to antibiotics, and treatment-related factors like the quantity and dosage of drugs, frequency of dosing, and length of treatment. Routine *H. pylori* testing following an attempt to treat the infection is not recommended in simple cases or after the first ulcer is detected. This is because the remission of symptoms in duodenal ulcer disease has been shown to be a reliable indicator of effective *H. pylori* eradication. To aid in the choice of an alternative treatment approach, the status of *H. pylori* and its antimicrobial resistance to metronidazole and clarithromycin should be assessed following the healing of a complex ulcer or in the event of an ulcer relapse. The efficacy of retreatment is more affected by post-treatment resistance than by pretreatment resistance during the initial course of treatment. Thus, in general, medications that have been shown to be resistant to *H. pylori* should not be used in rescue therapy. After testing for resistance, selecting a retreatment plan is typically simple if resistance has only evolved to one drug class, such as imidazoles or macrolides, or if there is no evidence of resistance. In cases where imidazole resistance is evident, switching from imidazole to amoxicillin in PPI-triple therapy is typically a successful second-line treatment (Unge, 1999). If there is clarithromycin resistance, imidazole can be an effective second-line PPI triple treatment. Quadruple therapy is recommended as rescue therapy if the resistance pattern is unknown or if resistance to both macrolides and imidazoles has been demonstrated. Up to 70–75% of retreatments using triple therapy were found to have *H. pylori* eradication rates as low as 50% due to secondary imidazole resistance. In patients receiving critical care, gastric hemorrhage from ulceration and stress erosions is a significant complication that can result in up to 50–80% mortality as well as substantial morbidity. While the precise etiology of gastroduodenal mucosal lesions is still unknown, many factors have been found to contribute to their formation. Because randomized trials have shown beneficial results, prophylaxis with acid-suppressive, acid-neutralizing, or cytoprotective medicines has been widely suggested. Since the latest research suggests that the current incidence of clinically significant lesions maybe 5% or less, routine stress ulcer prophylaxis has been studied. As a result, stress ulcer prophylaxis is only recommended for people who are at elevated risk. The crucial preventive action is appropriate resuscitation, which aims to enhance oxygenation and the state of the heart. The risk variables that are linked to bleeding from stress ulcers are coagulopathy and respiratory failure.

Before considering the use of H2RAs, it is advisable to assess the intragastric pH. High-dose H2RA, preferably via continuous infusion, is more effective than placebo in preventing clinically significant bleeding in patients with hyperacidity. Antacids neutralize intragastric acid in a dose-dependent manner. Antacids should be administered every 1–2 hours for best effects (Washington and Wilson, 1986). If the time between doses is more than three hours, their effectiveness diminishes. Antacids containing aluminum hydroxide neutralize acid and bind pepsin and promote mucosal prostaglandin synthesis, which increases mucus and bicarbonate output and improves mucosal blood flow. Frequent antacid administration, ideally in conjunction with intragastric pH monitoring, is labor-intensive and frequently results in nasogastric tube obstructions. Antacid side effects can include constipation, diarrhea, hypophosphatemia, and hypermagnesemia. This is a simple saccharo-octasulfate aluminum salt having a little antacid effect. It binds pepsin and increases prostaglandin synthesis, which improves mucus layer, mucosal regeneration, and mucosal blood flow, much like aluminum-containing antacids do. About as effective as antacids in preventing bleeding from stress ulcers is sucralfate (4–6 g/day). Technical issues may arise during nasogastric tube administration.

7.12. Non-Steroidal Anti-Inflammatory Drugs

NSAIDs, or non-steroidal anti-inflammatory drugs, are a popular class of medications used to treat dysmenorrhea and musculoskeletal pain. They do not contain aspirin. Approximately 50% of NSAID users experience dyspepsia or stomach pain, and a large portion experience gastrointestinal problems like bleeding. The likelihood of these problems may rise by a factor of four to five, but the likelihood is largely influenced by patient risk factors like age, history of ulcer disease, etc., and the type of NSAID taken. While enteric-coated or buffered aspirin and NSAIDs are frequently more well accepted, they do not appear to lower the risks when administered via rectal. Up to 60% of NSAID-using patients have gastroduodenal lesions with limited clinical relevance, such as erosions and/or intramucosal hemorrhage. It is believed that the chance of developing a duodenal or stomach ulcer in patients on NSAID therapy is 5–20% and 2–3%, respectively. Up to 60% of patients may experience life-threatening consequences as a result of NSAID-induced gastrointestinal bleeding without any prior warning indications. The doctor should carefully weigh the benefits for each patient against the possible risks of ulcers and their complications. Acetylsalicylic acid is one of the NSAIDs with topical harmful effects that may contribute to its ulcer-causing potential. Since most NSAIDs are weak acids, non-ionized NSAIDs penetrate into epithelial cells across the cell membrane in an acidic environment. The ionization of the elevated intracellular pH causes intraepithelial trapping and accumulation. NSAIDs function by preventing the synthesis of pro-inflammatory peptides like prostacyclin and PGE2 by inhibiting cyclo-oxygenase (Khan et al., 2019). These prostanoids cause the mucosal microcirculation to vasodilate, increase the release of gastric mucus and bicarbonate, and limit the secretion of acid. There are two isoforms of cyclo-oxygenase (COX): COX-1, which has multiple physiological functions, such as preserving normal function in the GI and renal tracts, and COX-2, which is controlled by pro-inflammatory stimuli. Prostaglandins control the secretion of mucin and surface-active phospholipids, hence NSAIDs decrease the function of the mucus barrier. NSAIDs also prevent mucosal cell proliferation, which is essential for erosion or ulcer formation, and prostaglandin-mediated bicarbonate production from the stomach and duodenal mucosa. NSAIDs have the potential to cause microvascular ischemia, which could result in cellular components adhering to the vascular endothelium. Reduced blood flow and the buildup of active neutrophils may eventually cause ischemic cell damage that makes ulcers more likely. In animal models, NSAID-induced damage is enhanced by blocking the generation of nitric oxide (NO), whereas NSAID toxicity is decreased by NO donors. Given that inflammatory stimuli trigger the production of COX-2, it is probable that the inhibition of COX-2 is responsible for the anti-inflammatory benefit of NSAIDs, while the inhibition of COX-1 is primarily responsible for the side effects. Since most NSAIDs are not fully selective for COX-2, severe events resulting from undesired COX-1 effects are common.

In comparison to NSAIDs with a less favorable COX-2: COX-1 activity ratio, those with the strongest activity against COX-2 and the most favorable COX-2/COX-1 activity ratio will have anti-inflammatory activity and fewer side effects. The creation of COX-2 selective NSAIDs has been prompted by the identification of COX-2. NO is known to mediate mucosal defense and shares many characteristics with prostaglandins in the gastrointestinal system. The NO that is generated will be helpful because it will maintain the blood flow through the mucosa, prevent adhesion to the endothelium, and prevent neutrophil activation. When taken for several weeks, these NO-releasing NSAIDs have been proven to protect the gastroduodenal mucosa while having the same anti-inflammatory effects as native NSAIDs. There is a minimal correlation between mucosal lesions and symptoms among NSAID users. While about 25% of patients taking NSAIDs report having stomach pain, NSAID-associated ulcers frequently go unnoticed. The symptoms are a poor indicator of problems related to NSAID use. Less than 1% of chronic NSAID users experience potentially fatal consequences within three to six months of use, although 10 to 30% of them develop peptic ulcers during that time. Many individuals with dyspepsia benefit from the recommendation to take NSAIDs with meals, even if there is not much data to support it. Studies on the withdrawal of NSAIDs in the old have shown that acetaminophen, another painkiller, works just as well in place of NSAIDs for up to two-thirds of those who take them chronically. Reducing the rate of clinically relevant problems like bleeding has not shown to be beneficial, despite efforts to reduce the harmful effects of NSAIDs by enteric coating and the development of slow-release formulations. The lowest effective dosage, the shortest duration, and the use of an NSAID with minimal risk of major gastrointestinal problems are advised if NSAIDs are actually necessary. Individuals over the age of 65 or 70, those with a history of complicated ulcer disease, those taking stronger NSAIDs at higher dosages, those taking aspirin concurrently to prevent myocardial infarction or stroke, and those exhibiting other clinical indicators of poor general health such as hospitalization or a history of renal or cardiac disease are among the patients who are more likely to experience serious ulcer complications. Infection with *H. pylori* does not increase the risk of bleeding in people on NSAIDs. It has been proposed that the interplay between *H. pylori* and NSAIDs in mucosal prostaglandin synthesis explains why ulceration is not caused by an additive impact. Many studies compare variations in the amount of mucosal lesions or blood loss in the feces, but few have assessed clinically reliable goals like bleeding, hospitalization rates, and mortality. In long-term clinical research, erosions should not be taken into account when evaluating the effectiveness of any preventive medication because they do not result in problems.

Because they affect the mucosal defense and repair processes, NSAIDs pose a risk to the integrity of the mucosa. It is not recommended to provide NSAIDs to all patients to prevent gastrointestinal effects, but high-risk patients should always be given extra care when using these drugs. It seems that the presence of acid is a requirement for NSAID-induced damage to the gastroduodenal mucosa. Research on animals has demonstrated that the extent and length of acid-inhibition play a critical role in averting damage to the mucosa of the stomach.

The main causes of emesis have been clustered into categories based on the principal emetic route in order to determine which medications are most effective against various forms of nausea and vomiting. Pharmacological selectivity is crucial for analyzing the processes and mechanisms that lead to vomiting in response to medications and diseases. It can be said that five primary stimulus types can cause nausea and vomiting, and each stimulus can work on many pathways.

These include: (a) Toxic chemicals, including medications, in the gut lumen excite primarily vagal afferents that project to the brainstem area postrema (AP) and nucleus tractus solitarius (NTS), which in turn causes emesis (Babic and Browning, 2014). (b) The area postrema, a circumventricular organ at the caudal extremity of the fourth ventricle floor where the blood–brain barrier (Figure 7.1) is relatively permeable, is directly stimulated by ingested toxic materials, including drugs or endogenous agents, and its outputs cause emesis. (c) Pathological conditions that either directly or indirectly activate pathways, such as hypertrophic pyloric stenosis, gastritis, or other visceral organ diseases including renal failure or myocardial infarction. (d) A stimulus triggers the emetic reflex inside the central nervous system, such as panic, brain damage, or an abrupt increase in intracranial pressure.

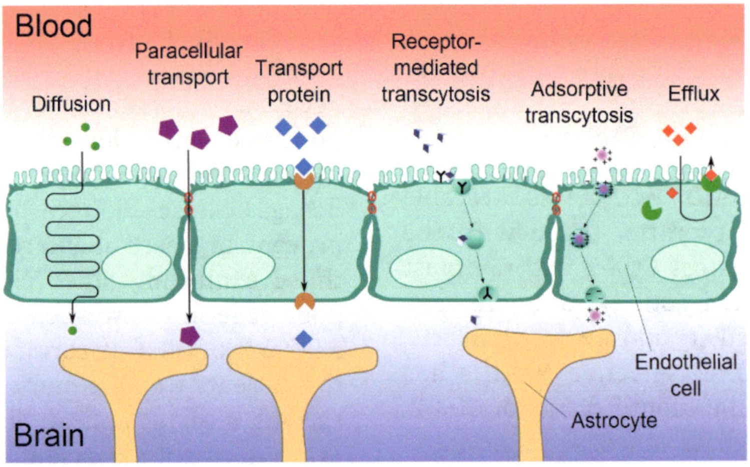

Figure 7.1. *Blood–brain barrier.*

Source: https://upload.wikimedia.org/wikipedia/commons/c/c6/Blood-brain_barrier_transport_en.png, Creative Commons License.

7.13. Addressing Emetic Reflex

The emetic reflex is triggered by a disruption of the vestibular system, such as motion sickness or Menière's illness (Cuomo-Granston and Drummond, 2010). Since head position affects sensitivity to the emetic drug apomorphine, which works on the AP, experimental research in humans has suggested that the vestibular system may also alter the sensitivity of the brainstem emetic pathways. The upper intestine is a primary region for detecting emetic signals. Vagal nerve afferents are primarily used in this area to transmit to the brainstem NTS, which in turn triggers emesis. The hepatic vagal afferents or the AP may detect stimuli through neuronal connections with the NTS. It is believed that cytotoxic anticancer medications cause free radicals to be produced in the gastrointestinal mucosa, which in turn causes enterochromaffin (EC) cells to emit 5-hydroxytryptamine (5-HT). The vagal nerve afferent terminals are located close to the EC cells; thus, the released 5-HT easily activates the 5-HT3 receptors on these terminals. The 5-HT3 receptor may play a major role in sensitizing the vagus nerve to other excitatory compounds, such as substance P, that are released from the EC cells or that are produced later on during the anti-cancer treatment. However, this process may also be the cause of emesis. Severe forms of nausea and vomiting could be the outcome. Treatment with 5-HT3 receptor antagonists can usually stop emesis during the first 24 hours; if the emesis is severe, as it does after high-dose cisplatin, adding a corticosteroid is advised. The latter have unknown methods of action, but the most likely one is that they decrease edema at an emetic-sensitive site and prevent the production of emetogenic chemicals by inhibiting eicosanoid metabolism. It is impossible to rule out corticosteroid non-genomic effects. Selective or non-selective dopamine D2 receptor antagonists may also help with mild cases of emesis. This activity suggests that the anti-cancer therapy produces emetogens, which function not only within the gut (via the 5-HT3 receptor) but also in the bloodstream to stimulate D2 receptors in the area postrema and/or on NTS neurons projecting into the area postrema, even though they are frequently less effective than 5-HT3 receptor antagonists. A similar mechanism is believed to function during radiation targeted at the abdominal regions, where the vomiting is susceptible to suppression by antagonists of the 5-HT3 receptor and, to a lesser degree, by antagonists of the D2 receptor.

Other exogenously delivered medications also have the ability to cause vomiting. Certain substances are believed to cause irritation to the gastrointestinal tract, which in turn causes the EC cells to release 5-HT and activate the 5-HT3 receptors on the vagal afferent nerve terminals. Clinical and/or animal trials that demonstrate emesis can be prevented by specific 5-HT3 receptor antagonism and, in certain cases, by abdominal vagotomy in animals support this hypothesis. These medications include phosphodiesterase IV enzyme inhibitors (rolipram), cytokines like interferon or interleukin 2, certain anti-infective regimens for HIV patients, pyrogallol-induced free radical generation, and overdoses of theophylline, acetaminophen/diphenhydramine/aspirin combination, and colchicine. The processes underlying the emesis induced by several other drugs remain unclear due to a lack of relevant studies or inconsistent evidence acquired following the injection of selective 5-HT3 receptor antagonists, such as morphine. Emesis induced by certain drugs may be inhibited by 5-HT3 or dopamine D2 receptor antagonism. This suggests that a toxin or drug in circulation may be able to induce emesis by activating D2 receptors in the area postrema as well as by releasing 5-HT from the gut. Nevertheless, given their capacity to prevent emesis induced by specific types of brain injury, 5-HT3 receptor antagonists may also, under some unique conditions, suppress central processes of emesis. It is evident that some drugs work directly through the area postrema and/or NTS dendrites and these types of emesis are resistant to inhibition by 5-HT3 receptor antagonism. Examples of such medications include loperamide, an opioid receptor agonist that causes emesis and is not affected by dopamine D2 or 5-HT3 antagonism but is diminished by naloxone and eliminated by area postrema ablation. The gastric prokinetic drug and the 5-HT4 receptor agonist cisapride may have no effect on vomiting in this situation, while 5-HT3 receptor antagonism reduces or eliminates it. Similar to the 5-HT3 receptor mechanism in the etiology of emesis in cancer patients undergoing cytotoxic therapy and with the symptoms of pruritis in patients with cholestatic disease, there may be a causal association between 5-HT and the symptoms of emesis and pruritis in patients with uremia. It has been proposed that the various combinations of emesis and/or pruritis rely, in part, on the source of 5HT but, mostly on the development of other sensory nerve irritants. Therefore, the primary function of 5-HT3 receptors is to increase the sensitivity of nerve endings to the excitatory effects of other drugs. Therefore, the expression of 5-HT3 receptor activity depends on a specific visceral afferent nerve accessibility to pathogenic concentrations of 5-HT and other excitatory compounds like histamine and substance P.

7.14. Obstruction

In cases of partial obstruction, especially those associated with motor disorders or drug-induced nausea, it is important to suppress the nausea with medications that promote aboral gastrointestinal propulsion. The effectiveness of these treatments varies, though. By partially activating the 5-HT4 receptor and promoting the cholinergic motor pathways within the peristaltic reflex, cisapride, and metoclopramide increase gut motility; their affinity and lack of selectivity for the 5-HT4 receptor are well-documented. Metoclopramide is used, for instance, in a continuous subcutaneous infusion to treat narcotic bowel syndrome (Farmer et al., 2017). Domperidone, a selective D2 receptor antagonist, lacks a definite intrinsic ability to induce gastrointestinal motility. Its limited blood-brain barrier penetration means that it typically does not cause the extrapyramidal adverse effects associated with metoclopramide. It is thought to increase gastrointestinal motility by eliminating a dopamine-mediated inhibitory effect on the gut. Domperidone relieves gastric stasis since it antagonizes D2 receptors and subsequently exhibits anti-emetic action. It is unclear if there are any other disorders where the gut experiences an improper dopamine surge, although they might include dyspepsia or diseases linked to mental stress. Drugs that increase gastrointestinal motility should be avoided in cases of total bowel obstruction as the gut may attempt to commence propulsive action against the obstruction. This generates a cycle of distension, secretion, and motor activity, causing discomfort, intestinal retropulsion, and vomiting. Antiemetic and analgesic medications, as well as decompression techniques, are used as forms of treatment, although surgery is frequently the main course of action. The D2 receptor antagonist haloperidol, the H1 receptor antagonist cyclizine, or the combination of both processes through the use of phenothiazine are examples of anti-emetic medications.

7.15. Other Medications and Side Effects

Chlorpromazine is used to treat terminal disease-related nausea and vomiting (Davis and Walsh, 2000). Sedation and antimuscarinic symptoms are other side effects. It is not advised in cases of phaeochromocytoma, bone marrow depression, or CNS depressants-induced coma. Phenazine is used to treat severe nausea and vomiting. Perphenazine has a similar side as chlorpromazine, but it is less sedative; extrapyramidal responses are more common. Prochlorperazine is used to treat a variety of ailments, including severe nausea and vomiting. Prochlorperazine is less sedating than chlorpromazine, but it has additional side effects and contraindications, including a higher frequency of extrapyramidal responses, including dystonia. Trifluoperazine is used in cases of extreme nausea, and vomiting. The same adverse events and contraindications apply to chlorpromazine, except for decreased sedation, hypotension, hypothermia, and antimuscarinic side effects. Extrapyramidal symptoms, particularly dystonia and akathisia, are more common. Domperidone is used to treat functional dyspepsia, acute nausea, and vomiting after cytotoxic or radiation treatment. Extrapyramidal side effects (rare), renal impairment and pregnancy are additional contraindications. Domperidone is not advised for chronic administration or the prevention of postoperative vomiting. Antagonists of histamine H1 receptors are Dimenhydrinate, Cinnarizine, Cyclizine, Meclozine, and Promethazine. Histamine H1 receptor antagonists are used to treat vomiting at levels that have been established and confirmed by primarily antagonistic interactions with histamine H1 receptors in vestibular and brainstem nuclei. Antiemetic, therapeutic, and side-effects are exerted via other non-selective activities.

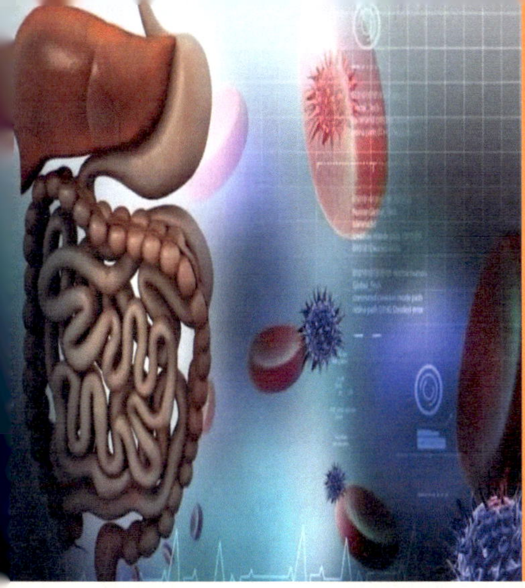

Chapter 8

INFECTIONS OF THE GASTROINTESTINAL SYSTEM

Contents

8.1. Introduction

Species of Aeromonas are found in soil and water sources all over the world. A major cause of infection is exposure to polluted water, but it can also happen from eating contaminated foods including dairy, meat, and fruit. The intestinal flora of humans does not include aeromonads. Because they are rarely isolated from the feces of asymptomatic individuals, it was formerly thought that they were nonpathogenic. Gastroenteritis in infants and adults will be due to weakened immune systems. This is because the organism can be recovered from the stool of symptomatic patients when other pathogens are not present, and the organism subsequently completely responds to antibiotic therapy. Though other species may also be involved, humans are frequently affected by gastrointestinal disorders caused by the motile *Aeromonas hydrophila* and *Aeromonas sobria* (Moyer, 1987).

8.2. Infections

The common seasons for gastrointestinal Aeromonas infections are late spring, early summer, and early fall, frequently, children are impacted. Mild diarrheal disease was reported, occasionally with nausea, vomiting, and cramping abdominal pain. In 15–20% of cases, a severe dysentery-like disease with fecal leukocytes and bloody/ mucoid diarrhea follows. From an endoscopic perspective, this resembles chronic idiopathic inflammatory bowel disease. A small percentage of patients have subacute, chronic diarrhea that lasts for months or years. Because the symptoms are persistent, they may clinically resemble chronic idiopathic inflammatory bowel disease. Mucosal edema and loss of vascular pattern are among the endoscopic observations.

Severe pancolitis that resembles fulminant ulcerative colitis has been reported. The histologic characteristics typically seen in acute colitis include neutrophilic infiltrates in the lamina propria, cryptitis, and crypt abscesses. Focal architectural distortion and ulceration may be observed in certain instances. Ischemic colitis, chronic idiopathic inflammatory bowel disease, and other infectious colitides are included in the differential diagnosis. Stool cultures are essential for diagnosis, and you might need to use a certain selective medium. In cases where a patient exhibits architectural distortion along with persistent symptoms or macroscopic characteristics similar to chronic idiopathic inflammatory bowel disease, distinguishing between Aeromonas infection and ulcerative colitis or Crohn's disease can be challenging. Exacerbations of idiopathic inflammatory bowel disease have been linked to Aeromonas. For these reasons, some researchers advise culturing for Aeromonas in all patients with refractory chronic inflammatory bowel disease and in individuals whose first presentation of chronic idiopathic inflammatory bowel disease is suspected, especially in children. As with many infections of the gastrointestinal tract, Aeromonas infection lacks distinct histologic indications, but the surgical pathologist must understand that this is one of the bacteria that can most closely mimic chronic idiopathic inflammatory bowel disease. *Edwardsiella tarda* and *Plesiomonas shigelloides* are comparable freshwater bacteria. They are thought to induce a similar clinical, macroscopic, and histologic spectrum of disease, while being less frequently isolated than Aeromonas species.

8.3. Cholera

The causal agent of cholera, an important cause of watery diarrhea and dysentery that can result in severe dehydration, an imbalance in electrolytes, and death in a matter of hours, is *Vibrio cholerae*, more especially the toxic 01 strain. The majority of cases in the US involve people who have visited endemic or epidemic regions. Consuming raw or undercooked seafood, especially shellfish, is the primary cause of most diseases. Severe gastroenteritis can also be brought on by other Vibrios, such as non-01 strains of *V. cholera* (Figure 8.1), *V. hollisae*, and *V. parahaemolyticus* (Bhunia, 2018).

Cholera is characterized by an onset of diarrhea that is typically watery and very rarely bloody. Other symptoms include fever, cramping in the muscles, vomiting, and stomach pain. Bloody diarrhea, fecal leukocytes, and spread to extraintestinal locations are common symptoms of strains other than toxigenic O1 *V. cholerae*; nonetheless, the clinical manifestations caused by toxigenic *V. cholerae* O1 and other Vibrios may be identical. Immunocompromised patients are especially vulnerable to infection; patients with underlying liver disease, those who have had a partial or complete gastrectomy, and those with disorders affecting iron metabolism are also susceptible to serious Vibrio infections. Toxigenic *V. cholerae* O1 is a non-invasive pathogen that causes little to no histologic alterations in the stomach, regardless of how severe the disease is. Some researchers have reported non-specific observations include depletion of small bowel mucus, surface epithelial alterations caused by degeneration, and an elevation of lamina propria mononuclear cells. These Gram-negative bacteria are a global cause of diarrhea and are often isolated stool bacteria in the United States. Campylobacter is frequently linked to consuming raw milk, contaminated water, and undercooked chicken. It is a common veterinary pathogen that can infect when they come into contact with diseased animals. Along with *C. coli* and *C. laridis*, *Campylobacter jejuni* is frequently linked to food-borne gastroenteritis; in contrast, immunosuppressed individuals and homosexual men are more likely to have *C. fetus* and other uncommon species. All age groups are susceptible to campylobacter infection, although infants, kids, and young adults are most frequently afflicted. HIV-positive patients have a greater incidence than the total population, and they are more likely to have severe, persistent, recurring infections. Most infections diminish on their own, particularly in immunocompetent patients; immunocompromised patients or those with long-lasting, severe, or extensive infections may need antibiotics and supportive treatment. Campylobacter infection can lead to the development of many autoimmune diseases, such as reactive arthropathy, Henoch-Schonlein purpura, and Guillain-Barre syndrome, which can be linked to Campylobacter in as many as 40% of cases. Infections with Campylobacter can potentially exacerbate underlying chronic idiopathic inflammatory bowel disease.

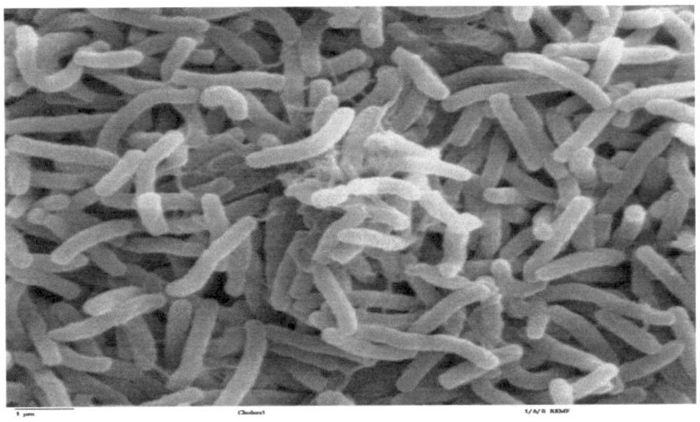

Figure 8.1. *Vibrio cholerae.*

Source: https://upload.wikimedia.org/wikipedia/commons/9/9d/Cholera_bacteria_SEM.jpg, Creative Commons License.

Fever, tiredness, gastric discomfort, and watery diarrhea frequently contain blood and leukocytes are typical symptoms. For many patients, the main symptom may be abdominal pain. There may be varying degrees of headache, myalgias, tenesmus, nausea, and vomiting. In one to two weeks, symptoms usually go away, but relapses are frequent. Friable colonic mucosa with accompanying erythema and bleeding are among the endoscopic findings. There could be inflammatory exudates and ulceration. Rare cases have been documented of segmental colitis or pancolitis that macroscopically resembles ulcerative colitis. Nonetheless, a colonoscopy might not be significant. The infectious colitis that is commonly seen on histologic examination include cryptitis, crypt abscesses, surface epithelial destruction, and a neutrophilic infiltrate in the lamina propria. There may be visible edema and superficial mucosal erosion along with bleeding. Colon biopsy reveals that *C. jejuni* is present in about 20% of individuals with the focal active colitis pattern of inflammation (Bhaijee et al., 2015). This finding was made using molecular approaches. Generally, crypt architecture is generally conserved, but there are isolated instances of mild crypt deformation, crypt epithelial injury, and crypt loss. In the small bowel, comparable morphologic results may be observed. Other infections including Salmonella, Shigella, and Aeromonas that cause acute infectious or self-limited colitis are primarily included in the differential diagnosis. Chronic idiopathic inflammatory bowel disease can be mistaken for Campylobacter colitis when crypt distortion is observed. Stool culture is a crucial diagnostic technique; additional options include molecular assays, darkfield stool examination, and serologic investigations. *Helicobacter pylori* is a spirillar or coccoid Gram-negative bacterium that causes stomach infections. It was formerly known as *Campylobacter pyloridis*. Although the prevalence of *H. pylori* (HP) infection is declining, partly as a result of eradication efforts, it is still one of the most widespread bacterial diseases globally, affecting an estimated 50% of the global population. The majority of cases are caused by person-to-person transmission through the fecal-oral, oral-oral, and gastric-oral pathways; however, acquisition through zoonotic or environmental sources cannot be ruled out. Young age and low socioeconomic level are risk factors.

8.4. The Morphological Changes in Gastritis

Many gastrointestinal conditions, such as gastric adenocarcinoma, peptic ulcers, atrophic gastritis, chronic gastritis, and lymphomas of the mucosa-associated lymphoid tissue (MALT) type are linked to *H. pylori* infection. Gastritis linked to *H. pylori* in patients may manifest as dyspepsia, epigastric discomfort, nausea, vomiting, and gastrointestinal hemorrhage. However, many diseased individuals do not show any symptoms. The presence or intensity of histologic findings does not always correspond well with endoscopic findings. Mucosal granularity, aberrant vascular pattern, and erythema are examples of the highly non-specific mucosal alterations. Mucosal nodules may be observed, particularly in young patients, and they may be associated with lymphoid hyperplasia. The fundic and cardiac mucosa are frequently involved, but the antrum is more frequently impacted. Chronic, active gastritis is the inflammatory pattern frequently linked to HP infection. It is characterized by a neutrophil infiltration of the glandular epithelium and a mononuclear cell infiltrate in the lamina propria, which is rich in plasma cells. Within the inflammatory infiltrate, scattered eosinophils are also frequently seen. Frequently observed features include lymphoid clusters, which can have variable germinal centers and prominent intraepithelial lymphocytosis. The mucosal architecture is often largely intact; however, the epithelium may exhibit a serrated appearance, reactive nuclear alterations, or mucus depletion. There is typically no relationship between the quantity of organisms detected and the degree of inflammation. The use of proton pump inhibitors and anti-HP drugs may cause the bacteria to migrate closer to the corpus and reduce the amount of inflammation. The presence of lymphoid follicles and the chronic inflammatory infiltrate resolve more slowly, and these alterations typically manifest a year or longer following the removal of the organism.

8.5. Helicobacter pylori (HP)

Invasive species are rarely observed; they live in the pits as well as at the luminal surface. HP can have a very patchy distribution. The spirilla bacteria may change into coccoid forms, which resemble mucus droplets, non-pathogenic bacteria, or other species like coccidians or fungal spores (Lamps, 2010). Since coccoid forms are linked with spirilla forms, even though the exact clinical significance of coccoid forms is unknown, the diagnosis of HP infection when only coccoid forms are present should be treated carefully. For a thorough assessment of the HP infection state, many research sources advise obtaining some biopsies, one from the lesser and one from the larger curvature, and one or more from the gastric corpus. While there is ongoing debate on the necessity of specific stains for HP diagnosis, most research experts agree that staining is required, especially in cases where the patient has received prior treatment, the infection is patchy, or intestinal metaplasia is present. Giemsa and silver impregnation stains like the Warthin-Starry or Steiner are useful stains. The latter can be mixed with hematoxylin and eosin (H&E) and Alcian blue to produce the triple or Genta stain, which also makes it possible to assess the morphology of the stomach. Although the process of silver impregnation stains is more costly and technically complex, the microbes are easily recognized by this method because they appear large and stain a dark black color. Although they are less frequently utilized, HP can also be detected using the fluorescent acridine orange stain and Gram stain. The immunostain, however, might react negatively with other species of Helicobacter. Other non-erosive, non-specific causes of gastritis, such as autoimmune gastritis, Crohn's disease, infectious gastroenteritis, adverse drug reactions, and the lymphocytic gastritis linked to celiac disease, are the main differential diagnosis options. It is important to differentiate MALT lymphoma from *H. pylori*-related gastritis if there is an unusually thick inflammatory infiltrate.

8.6. Other Pathogens

A neoplastic process is supported by architectural degradation, lymphocyte infiltration into the submucosa, and multiple lymphoepithelial lesions (Businello et al., 2020). However, gene rearrangement investigations may be necessary to confirm the diagnosis. The morphology of the organism is necessary to differentiate *H. pylori* from contaminating oropharyngeal flora, which can likewise stain on non-specific histochemical stains. It needs to be differentiated from other, less frequent species of Helicobacter. When testing for antibiotic susceptibility is required, the most common method, which is also the most difficult, is to culture the organism. Urease tests, such as CLO, are quick, cheap, and have sensitivity and specificity that are similar to histology. Breath tests that measure carbon isotope excretion are quick, accurate, and non-invasive; but the costs are high, the tests are not commonly available, and certain procedures include a small amount of radiation exposure. Serologic studies are low cost and have good sensitivity and specificity. In the absence of treatment, a positive result suggests active infection; nevertheless, positive serologic results might last long after the bacteria have been eradicated. There are assays for molecular detection as well, but they are not common. The less common Helicobacter species *H. heilmannii* (HH), formerly known as *Gastrospirillum hominis*, is linked to animal contact, especially with dogs, cats, cattle, and pigs. It can infect both adults and children and causes symptoms akin to those of HP. Rarely, *H. heilmannii* infection has been linked to the development of ulcers, especially when non-steroidal anti-inflammatory drug use is present. Co-infection with HH and HP is well-documented. While the gastritis resulting from HH and HP share the same morphology, the former is frequently more localized, less severe, and linked to fewer organisms. HH infections are typically limited to the antrum. Some researchers have linked HH to edema, increased intracytoplasmic mucin, vascular dilatation, and foveolar hyperplasia. Less frequently, HH is linked to intestinal metaplasia, gastric adenocarcinoma, and MALT lymphoma.

Compared to HP, *H. heilmannii* is more densely coiled and longer. The same histochemical stains used to detect HP can also be used to detect *H. heilmannii*. *H. heilmannii* is immunopositive for the anti-*H. pylori* immunohistochemistry stains. Although *H. felis* is known to rarely infect humans, it is unknown if this can lead to gastritis. Other intermittently occurring Helicobacter species include *H. rappini*, which also causes diarrhea; *H. canis* and *H. winghamensis*, which cause gastroenteritis; and *H. cinaedi*, which are thought to cause Campylobacter-like lower GI symptoms in immunocompromised patients. These species have one or more animal hosts. Since these organisms must be isolated using specialized microbiological methods, little is known about how common infection is in humans and how they relate to their animal reservoirs. These Gram-negative bacteria are common in areas with inadequate sanitation and are spread by contaminated food and water. They are also a major contributor to traveler's diarrhea and occasional food poisoning in developed countries. Meat, milk, eggs, and egg products, and sometimes vegetables and fruits can harbor salmonella, which can withstand freezing, drying, and partial cooking. Infections can spread through food handlers, and infections can also come from animals. Individuals with AIDS are more likely to get Salmonella infections, and those with low stomach acidity are more susceptible to salmonellosis. Even while supportive care and medications can usually treat most Salmonella infections in wealthy nations, intestinal infections can lead to septicemia. This is especially dangerous for individuals who are old, very young, have compromised immune systems, or have comorbid diseases. Antibiotics are especially crucial for newborns, elderly patients, immunocompromised individuals, patients with heart problems, and patients with indwelling prostheses. Delayed therapy is linked to increased mortality. In the gall bladder, a chronic carrier condition has hardly been reported. It is interesting to note that those who have schistosomiasis also have a higher chance of developing salmonellosis since the bacterium enters the parasites and grows there, acting as a nidus for subsequent infections.

8.7. Typhoid and GI Disease

Typhoid fever is commonly caused by *S. typhi*, (Figure 8.2) while *S. paratyphi* can also induce a similar clinicopathologic spectrum (Khan et al., 2006). Gastroenteritis is typically caused by nontyphoid species, such as *S. enteritidis*, *S. typhimurium*, and *S. paratyphi*. Typhoid fever patients usually present with fever, headache, abdominal pain, and sometimes beginning constipation. Leukopenia, delirium, hepatosplenomegaly, and an abdominal rash known as rose spots are all rather prevalent. In the second or third week of infection, diarrhea usually starts out watery but can become severe enough to cause perforations and extensive bleeding in the gastrointestinal tract. The ileum, appendix, and right colon exhibit the disease, but any level of the alimentary tract may be affected. The intestinal wall is thickened, and elevated (raised) nodules that resemble hyperplastic Peyer's patches can be observed. As the disease advances, it is usual to develop ulceration and necrosis, ovoid ulcers, and linear ulcers covering Peyer's patches. Typhoid fever can be made more complicated by perforation and toxic megacolon, and there is sometimes suppurative mesenteric lymphadenitis. The mucosa may occasionally be either extremely normal or slightly edematous and inflamed. Typhoid fever usually causes a mononuclear inflammatory infiltrate. After Peyer's patches hyperplasia, the surrounding epithelium becomes acutely inflamed. Eventually, macrophages, which are typically undetectable, infiltrate, and destroy the lymphoid follicles, sometimes in combination with plasma cells and lymphocytes. Necrosis starts in the Peyer's patch, moves to the mucosa nearby, and finally ulcerates there. Usually deep, the base of the ulcers is at the level of the muscularis propria. Granulomas are uncommon. There is also architectural deformation that resembles Crohn's disease or ulcerative colitis.

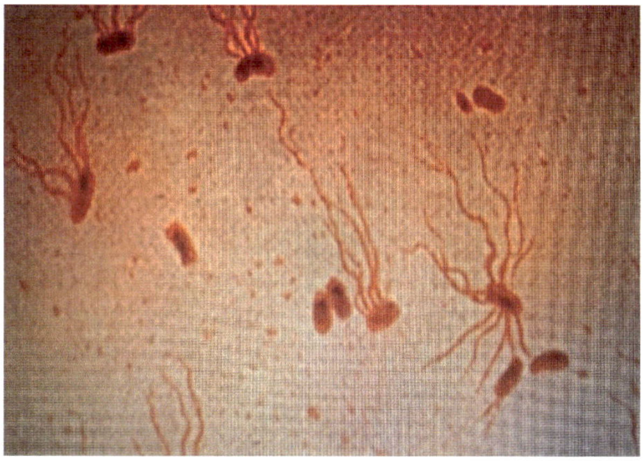

Figure 8.2. *Salmonella typhi.*

Source: https://upload.wikimedia.org/wikipedia/commons/7/74/SalmonellaTyphiFlagellarStain.jpg, Creative Commons License.

8.8. Salmonella and Shigella

Salmonella species that are not typhoid typically manifest 8–48 hours after consuming contaminated food or water, causing a less severe gastroenteritis with vomiting, nausea, fever, and watery diarrhea. Megacolon or severe bloody diarrhea are uncommon symptoms of non-typhoid species (Anderson, 2017). Colon perforation in children under the age of one year is frequently caused by non-typhoid Salmonellae. The common but less severe indications include mucosal erythema, bleeding, ulceration, and exudates. Sometimes the mucosa is either normal or only slightly hyperemic and edematous, and lesions might be localized. Usually, the histologic characteristics are similar to those of enterocolitis or non-specific acute infectious-type colitis. Severe instances may exhibit fibrinous exudates, tiny microthrombi, cryptitis, mucus depletion, and occasionally severe crypt deformation. There is some histological overlap between typhoid and non-typhoid species. Typhoid fever patients should be aware that they could not have the typical ulcer covering a Peyer's patch and instead have histologic characteristics more in line with acute self-limited colitis. Individuals with salmonellosis that is not typhoid may get severe colitis that involves ulceration and transmural involvement. In addition to ulcerative colitis (UC) and Crohn's disease, the differential diagnosis of typhoid fever also includes yersiniosis and other enteric bacterial infections. When architectural distortion is evident, there may be a substantial histologic overlap between chronic idiopathic inflammatory bowel disease and salmonellosis. Clinically, compared to other comparable intestinal pathogens, *S. typhi* infections require a longer incubation period (10–15 days). Compared to other enteric infections and idiopathic inflammatory bowel disease, typhoid fever frequently has fewer neutrophils, while salmonellosis rarely has granulomas. Significant crypt distortion is typically more noticeable in ulcerative colitis, though it has been noted in certain typhoid fever cases as well. In addition to other causes of chronic idiopathic inflammatory bowel disease, the differential diagnosis of non-typhoid Salmonella includes additional causes of acute self-limited infectious colitis.

If chronic idiopathic inflammatory bowel disease (IBD) already exists, a Salmonella infection may make it worse. Stool and/or blood cultures combined with the correct biochemical tests for species identification can be very helpful in determining the differential diagnosis between Salmonella infections that are not typhoid fever and those that are. Globally, Shigella, a type of invasive, pathogenic Gram-negative bacilli, is a leading cause of infectious diarrhea. Shigellosis is endemic in tropical and subtropical regions of Africa, Southern Asia, and Central America; it is particularly prevalent in underdeveloped countries with inadequate sanitation. Four species are part of the Shigellae family: *S. dysenteriae*, *S. boydii*, and *S. sonnei*. While reports of *S. sonnei* and *S. flexneri* are growing in the US, *Shigella dysenteriae* is the prevalent and virulent species that is isolated. Transmission can occur by food or water, but it can also be transmitted from person to person through the oral or fecal route. Out of all the enteric Gram-negative bacteria, it has the highest incidence of infectivity, and ingesting just 10–100 organisms can cause symptoms. Males who identify as homosexual, underweight patients, and children under the age of six are frequently affected. Shigellosis outbreaks are frequently observed in prisons, and day-care centers and are linked to unsanitary living conditions and overcrowding. Shigella is sexually contagious, and the prevalence of sexually transmitted shigellosis is rising among American homosexual men. The microscopic and macroscopic characteristics of shigellosis may closely resemble those of chronic idiopathic inflammatory bowel disease, much like salmonellosis does. The symptoms typically appear 12 to 50 hours after consuming contaminated food or water. The first symptoms are constitutional, such as fever, malaise, and abdominal pain. The diarrhea usually starts off watery and then turns red, sometimes with pus or mucus, and sometimes with tenesmus. Serious dehydration, sepsis, perforation, toxic megacolon, Reiter's syndrome, reactive arthritis, and hemolytic-uremic syndrome are among the complications. The most common cause of dysentery and major complications is *S. dysenteriae*. Both *S. flexneri* and *S. sonnei* infections are often self-limited and severe, though recovery could take up to seven days.

The ileum may also be impacted, but the large bowel is usually affected severely on the distal left side (Brown and Adam, 2002). Distribution is frequently continuous at first and can resemble ulcerative colitis; as the disease improves, patchy involvement becomes more typical. The mucosa is hemorrhagic and edematous, and exudates have the potential to produce pseudomembranes. There are varying degrees of ulceration. The rectum typically has the most severe morphologic alterations. Early symptoms of acute infectious type colitis typically include ulceration, edema, mucin depletion, cryptitis, often superficial crypt abscesses, and superficial neutrophilic infiltration. Apthoid ulcers are sporadic and resemble Crohn's disease. Microthrombi are visible, and pseudomembranes resembling Clostridium difficile infections are rather common. Increased mucosal damage and a high concentration of neutrophils and mononuclear inflammatory cells in the lamina propria are signs of the disease progression. Shigellosis is well-characterized by architectural alterations that resemble idiopathic inflammatory bowel disease, such as crypt branching, crypt dilatation, and crypt distortion. Salmonella that is not typhoid and enteroinvasive *Escherichia coli* are the two main pathogens that are included in the differential diagnosis of early shigellosis. The colitis brought on by *C. difficile* may have similarities with pseudomembranous shigellosis; in this case, the *C. difficile* antigen test can be highly beneficial. Shigellosis can be very difficult to diagnose later in the disease, both endoscopically and histologically, from Crohn's disease or ulcerative colitis. The resolution of the differential diagnosis may be greatly aided by the clinical presentation, such as the sudden onset of symptoms. Due to the fastidious nature and rapid death of Shigella, stool cultures are crucial, and specimens should be swiftly injected into the proper culture plates. It could be important to incorporate multiple cultures. There are various molecular tests available for the detection of shigellosis.

8.9. E. coli and Other Pathogens

Regular stool cultures are unlikely to differentiate pathogenic strains from the usual gut flora, which means that these diseases are significantly underdiagnosed. The most prevalent Gram-negative human pathogen is *Escherichia coli*. If pathogenic *E. coli* stains are suspected, the clinical laboratory should be alerted so that they can look for them precisely and use serotyping and specific culture techniques on specialized agars. Because pathogenic *E. coli* strains frequently disappear from stool quickly, cultures should be obtained as soon as feasible. Both infantile diarrhea and traveler's diarrhea are caused by enterotoxigenic *E. coli* (ETEC) in developing countries (Gascon et al., 1993). While unsanitary environments are the common places for infections to emerge, developed countries have also reported significant food-borne epidemics. ETEC infections are spread through contaminated food and water. The most significant outbreaks in US history have involved semisoft cheese, involving contaminated processing water and machinery that affected multiple lots of cheese across multiple states. Also connected to transmission are fresh produce and seafood. Enterotoxins produced by these non-invasive *E. coli* result in secretory diarrhea. Watery diarrhea, akin to cholera, can occasionally be accompanied by vomiting, nausea, low-grade fever, diarrhea, headaches, and cramps in the abdomen.

Usually, symptoms start to show up one to two days after consumption. There are no human descriptions of the microscopic or gross pathology associated with Enteropathogenic *E. coli* (ETEC). Very slight histopathologic alterations that resemble cholera are observed in animal investigations. The majority of EPEC infections affect newborns and infants. The infection shares clinical similarities with enteroaggregative *E. coli* (EAEC), despite the O:H serotypes being distinct. Fever, malaise, vomiting, and mucoid, non-bloody diarrhea are all brought on by this non-invasive *E. coli*. The visual and microscopic pathology of EPEC has not been thoroughly documented; the diarrhea can be persistent, and in AIDS patients, chronic diarrhea and wasting have been linked to EPEC. EAEC is a major contributor to traveler's diarrhea and diarrhea in children, and there is growing recognition that these non-invasive *E. coli* can also cause chronic diarrhea and wasting in individuals with AIDS.

These organisms typically cause low-grade fever, vomiting, and non-bloody, non-mucoid, watery diarrhea. Dissemination with sepsis is not thought to occur because they are non-invasive. The majority of endoscopic findings are not significant. Histologic analysis reveals sloughing, nuclear pyknosis, cytoplasmic vacuolization, and epithelial disarray as degenerative surface epithelial cell alterations. Intraepithelial inflammatory cells are variable in presence, although neither architectural distortion nor cryptitis are present in conjunction. The most noticeable characteristic is a layer of adhering Gram-negative bacteria at the surface epithelium. Both loose and tight adhesion of the bacterium is possible. The histologic results may be readily overlooked at low light because they can be uneven and resemble an exaggerated brush border. Biopsies from infected patients may show no abnormalities at all under the microscope. Spirochetosis and normal mucosa are the primary entities in the differential diagnosis; unlike spirochetosis, the bacteria in EPEC and EAEC are not spirillar and are typically Gram-negative. Enteroinvasive *E. coli* or EIEC are relatively new pathogens, most likely due to earlier confusion with Shigella or other *E. coli* strains. Both genetically and in terms of clinical presentation and pathophysiology, they are similar to Shigella. Serologic assays show some cross-reactivity with Shigella antigens. These microorganisms are responsible for traveler's diarrhea and can be spread via contaminated cheese, water, and inter-personal contact. Tenesmus, fever, diarrhea, and cramping in the abdomen are some of the symptoms. In most cases, diarrhea is watery and may include blood or mucous. Leukocytes from feces are frequent. EIEC can cause systemic bacteremia and severe colitis because they can infiltrate the colonic epithelium; this can be especially problematic for AIDS patients (Peek et al., 2018). There is a lack of information regarding the pathophysiology of EIEC in humans. Given the resemblance of these organisms to Shigella, it is possible that the disease will mimic shigellosis.

The common symptoms of gastrointestinal diseases include intense cramping in the abdomen and bloody diarrhea. Fever is either non-existent or very mild compared to most infections. In certa*in situ*ations, non-bloody, watery diarrhea may appear first or develop before bloody diarrhea. Fecal leukocytes are present in only one-third of patients. The development of hemolytic-uremic syndrome is the dangerous side effect of Enterohemorrhagic *Escherichia coli* (EHEC), and older people and children are especially vulnerable to this potentially fatal condition. Some research studies suggest that using antibiotics to treat EHEC raises the chance of developing HUS. Patients usually have significant bleeding along with mural edema. Mucosa is degraded and ulcerated, and purulent discharge frequently oozes from wounds. Surgery may be necessary to remove edema if it becomes so severe as to impede flow or control bleeding. Usually, the colon is damaged. The histologic characteristics, which include significant edema and bleeding in the lamina propria and submucosa, together with concomitant acute inflammation of the mucosa, crypt withering, and lamina propria hyalinization, closely mimic ischemic colitis caused by other causes. Small caliber blood vessels may have microthrombi and occasionally pseudomembranes similar to antibiotic-associated pseudomembranous colitis. It is common to observe mucosal necrosis, which typically affects the upper mucosa while preserving the deeper crypts. The main differential diagnosis for EHEC is pseudomembranous colitis associated with *C. difficile* and ischemic colitis from other sources, from which EHEC may be histologically identical. Distinguishing between *E. coli* infection and ischemia can be aided by the patient's age, clinical history, and macroscopic abnormalities, which may include the likelihood of consuming contaminated food. To differentiate *C. difficile*-related colitis from EHEC, the *C. difficile* antigen test could be quite useful. *Klebsiella oxytoca* has recently been linked to a hemorrhagic colitis that is antibiotic-associated. Hemorrhagic, segmental, and devoid of pseudomembranes, this colitis is most prevalent in the colon. An antibiotic use history, particularly with penicillin's, may be helpful in differentiating this infection from EHEC. Stool cultures are very helpful in diagnosing infections; however, because microbiologic diagnosis necessitates screening on selective agar, ordinary stool cultures are unable to differentiate 0157:H7 from normal intestinal flora.

8.10. Yersinia and Gastroenteritis

In Western and Northern Europe, Yersinia is the cause of bacterial gastroenteritis. It is prevalent throughout the world; however, the prevalence of infection is increasing in both Europe and the US, a trend that could be attributed to improved detection techniques and increased awareness of Yersinia species as significant intestinal pathogens. The species that cause gastrointestinal ailments in humans are *Yersinia enterocolitica* (YE) and *Yersinia pseudotuberculosis* (YP) (Galindo et al., 2011).

Water and food can both spread Yersinia disease, and the bacteria is linked to fruit, meat, dairy products, and chocolate. Animals can also transmit infections. Infections linked to transplacental, hospital-acquired, transfusion-associated, and familial routes have also been extensively studied. These mesenteric lymphadenitis, colitis, ileitis, and appendicitis are all brought on by these Gram-negative coccobacilli. Many instances of granulomatous appendicitis are also caused by Yersinia infections. While yersiniosis typically diminishes on its own, there is ample evidence of persistent infections, such as chronic colitis. Serious infection is associated with risk factors such as iron overload, diabetes mellitus, cirrhosis, deferoxamine medication, and immunocompromised state. Sepsis, abscess formation, perforation, and blockage from inflammatory masses are among the complications that can arise from gastrointestinal infections. The most common age groups affected are young adults, children, and infants. Patients frequently arrive with bloody diarrhea, nausea, vomiting, and weight loss. Abdominal pain might be widespread, periumbilical, or in the right lower quadrant. Leukocytosis, pharyngitis, and fever are possible side effects. When symptoms persist for weeks or months, it is common for them to be misdiagnosed as chronic idiopathic inflammatory bowel disease. Yersinia infection is also linked to erythema nodosum and reactive polyarthritis. Individuals who have Yersinia-caused granulomatous appendicitis frequently exhibit symptoms that are similar to those of acute non-specific appendicitis.

Yersinia can infect any part of the intestine; however, it primarily affects the appendix, right colon, and ileum. The affected bowel features an edematous, swollen wall and nodular inflammatory masses that are concentrated on Peyer's patches. It is possible to observe mucosal friability, edema, loss of vascular pattern, and aphthoid ulcers. Exudates can appear occasionally. Depending on how they are distributed, the results could macroscopically resemble either ulcerative colitis or Crohn's disease. Similar to suppurative appendicitis, appendices are swollen and hyperemic, and perforation is frequent. Gross foci of necrosis may be seen in the lymph nodes. Inflammation patterns that are both granulomatous and suppurative are frequently combined. Epithelioid granulomas, hyperplastic Peyer's patches, and underlying ulceration are common indications of YE. YP-induced gastrointestinal infections are identified by granulomatous processes with central microabscesses, which are invariably accompanied by mesenteric adenopathy. The histological features of YE and YP infection share similar features. Both species can present with mucosal ulceration, lymph node involvement, transmural lymphoid aggregates, epithelioid granulomas with prominent lymphoid cuffing, and lymphoid hyperplasia. Transmural inflammation, granulomas, skip lesions, focal architectural distortion, fissuring, and/or aphthoid ulcers, and Crohn's disease may resemble each other. Follicular hyperplasia with sporadic microabscesses and epithelioid granulomas is frequently observed in mesenteric lymph nodes. However, non-specific reactive lymphoid hyperplasia in patients without granulomas or microabscesses is also often observed in infected individuals. Salmonella and mycobacteria are the two main infectious processes included in the differential diagnosis.

The differentiation between yersiniosis and mycobacterial infection is aided by acid-fast stains and culture findings. Differing clinical manifestations, together with higher neutrophil counts, microabscesses, and granulomas, could aid in differentiating between yersiniosis and salmonellosis. Gram staining is typically not useful in the diagnosis of Yersinia; however, serologic investigations, PCR assays, and cultures can be highly helpful in confirming the diagnosis. In the differential diagnosis of Yersinia-associated granulomatous appendicitis, sarcoidosis, foreign body reaction to fecal debris, and granulomatous inflammation (appendectomy) with antibiotic therapy are also considered. Although both Lymphogranuloma venereum and Cat Scratch Disease can cause comparable histologic characteristics and affect the mesenteric lymph nodes, they hardly ever involve the colon itself. Separating yersiniosis from Crohn's disease can be quite challenging. Yersinia DNA has been found in many chronic Crohn's disease cases; the relevance of this finding is still unknown (Leu et al., 2013).

8.11. Gastric Tuberculosis

In Western countries, tuberculosis can be attributed to various factors such as immigrant populations, and the AIDS epidemic. Tuberculosis is still prevalent in developing nations. Hematogenous spread from pulmonary or military disease, ingestion of contaminated milk, and swallowing infected sputum in cases of pulmonary tuberculosis are some of the mechanisms through which gastrointestinal tuberculosis can be contracted. The disease may first emerge as gastrointestinal symptoms rather than pulmonary ones, and AIDS patients are more likely than immunocompetent people to experience extrapulmonary tuberculosis symptoms. There is ample evidence of primary gastrointestinal tuberculosis in the absence of lung infection. Depending on the sites involved, gastrointestinal TB presents with different symptoms. The most often affected locations are the ileocecal and jejunoileal, most likely because of the lymphoid tissue prevalence in these regions. It is highly frequent to have associated mesenteric adenopathy. Less frequently, the rectum, duodenum, and ascending colon are involved. Although gastroesophageal, appendiceal, and anal/perianal involvement are uncommon, they should be highlighted for their potential consequences on pathophysiology. Compared to gastrointestinal involvement, peritoneal TB is slightly more prevalent and can result in both ascites and clinically severe adhesions.

Patients frequently experience non-specific symptoms, such as weight loss, fever, diarrhea, abdominal pain, or a palpable abdominal mass, regardless of the region of involvement. Additional symptoms include evidence of malabsorption, anorexia, night sweats, and malaise. There may also be GI hemorrhage. Anemia (Mild) and an increased erythrocyte sedimentation rate are examples of abnormalities in the laboratory. Stomach-related tuberculosis is the common cause of esophageal tuberculosis spread from nearby affected organs like lung or mediastinal lymph nodes. Hematemesis, odynophagia, dysphagia, and aspiration from a tracheo-esophageal fistula are typical clinical symptoms. The frequent symptom is ulcers, while reports of strictures are also seen. Patients with gastric TB typically report nausea, vomiting, and abdominal pain; this is mainly because of either gastric outlet obstruction or ulcerative lesions. Gastric tuberculosis is more prevalent than esophageal involvement (Rasheed et al., 2007). Anal TB is uncommon, although it is rather frequent in endemic areas. In addition to anal ulceration, fissures, fistulas, abscesses, and mass lesions that can resemble cancer, Crohn's disease, or other sexually transmitted infections, patients with anal/perianal tuberculosis frequently do not have lung disease. TB in the appendices is less common than ileocecal infection, appendix tuberculosis is frequently linked to it. It has also been extensively documented that periappendicular tuberculosis may be linked to peritoneal tuberculosis. Along with thickening mucosal folds and inflammatory nodules, the most common endoscopic finding is ulcers. Colon is commonly affected by a malformed ileocecal valve. It is possible to observe large inflammatory tumors called tuberculomas, which usually involve the ileocecum. Perforation, bleeding, and blockage are side effects. It is common to have mesenteric lymphadenopathy, which causes swollen and matted mesenteric lymph nodes. In certain instances, large foci of necrosis might be observed.

In advanced stages of the disease, the colon wall frequently becomes thicker and edematous, with lymphoid hyperplasia, fibrosis, and transmural inflammation. At the edge of the granulomas, lymphocytes are common, and occasionally, large cells are seen. Hyalinized and calcified lesions are common in older patients, and granulomas can be uncommon and challenging to locate.

Submucosal vascular inflammation is extensive, and areas of granulomatous inflammation are often covered by architectural deformation mimicking chronic idiopathic inflammatory bowel disease. Immunocompromised patients may have a high concentration of organisms, whereas immunocompetent individuals may have a low concentration and difficulty detecting them. The quantity of organisms may also vary depending on the age of the lesion and prior anti-tubercular medication. Although PCR assays are becoming more accessible, if the number of organisms is extremely low, sensitivity issues also arise with this technology. Purified protein derivative () tests can be useful; however, they are unreliable in individuals who are immunocompromised. Atypical mycobacteria like *M. bovis* and *M. kansasii* can produce comparable pathological results. Sarcoidosis, granulomatous drug responses, Behcet's disease, and other uncommon autoimmune diseases are included in the differential diagnosis, along with other granulomatous infections, particularly yersiniosis and fungal disease. The lymphoid cuffs that characterize yersiniosis granulomas are usually not caseating, although there may be a significant amount of histologic overlap. Acid-fast bacilli (AFB) and fungal stains, PCR tests, and culture may all be very helpful in narrowing down the differential diagnosis. Patients with sarcoidosis typically have high serum angiotensin-converting enzyme levels along with concurrent mediastinal or pulmonary lesions. Behcet's disease patients frequently experience mouth ulcers and/or skin rashes (Nair and Moots, 2017).

It can be challenging to differentiate between tuberculosis and Crohn's disease, especially in countries where the former is more prevalent. The presence of deep fistulas and fissures, transmural lymphoid clusters, linear rather than circumferential ulcers, and mucosal alterations of chronicity that are found away from areas of granulomatous inflammation are characteristics that represent Crohn's disease. Mucosal cobble stoning is frequently absent in tuberculosis. An additional complicating problem is that infliximab, a tumor necrosis factor alpha neutralizing drug used to treat rheumatoid arthritis and Crohn's disease, has lately been linked to tuberculosis. Given that the majority of these patients had extrapulmonary tuberculosis, the pattern of involvement in these patients is unusual. *Mycobacterium avium* is the mycobacterium found in GI tract isolates. It is uncommon in immunocompetent people, but it is typically observed in patients with AIDS and other immune-compromising diseases. It frequently appears later in the course of AIDS and is a sign of low CD4 counts. In AIDS patients, MAI (*Mycobacterium avium*-intracellular complex) infection continues to be the most prevalent systemic bacterial infection. Disseminated infections typically exhibit gastrointestinal involvement, with the lungs, bone marrow, liver, spleen, and lymph nodes frequently also being affected. Symptoms include weight loss, nausea, vomiting, and diarrhea; fever and night sweats are also common. Pain in the abdomen is an infrequent symptom. Although colonic and gastric involvement, as well as mesenteric adenopathy, may also be present, the small bowel is mainly affected. The most common macroscopic manifestation of MAI infection is a swollen, granular white mucosal nodule 2–4 mm in diameter with surrounding erythema. There have also been reports of mucosal hemorrhages and small ulcers. There are varying amounts of necrosis foci present in the swollen and solid mesenteric lymph nodes that are involved.

8.12. Enhanced Diagnosis

The patient's immunological status and the site of the lesion affect the histologic manifestations. Usually well-developed, epithelioid granulomas with or without necrosis are seen in immunocompetent patients.

Immunocompromised patient small intestinal biopsies typically reveal expanded villi due to a diffuse infiltration of histiocytes harboring bacilli, with no evidence of an inflammatory response aside from sporadic, poorly formed granulomas. The colon and other GI tract regions may exhibit comparable histiocytic infiltrates. Both PAS and GMS and Bacilli stain with acid-fast stains; any fast-dividing bacteria may stain positively on GMS stain, but this should not deter the pathologist from making an incorrect diagnosis of a fungal infection. Mycobacteria can also stain for keratin, actin, and desmin. Assays for PCR and culture may be very beneficial in the diagnosing process. In immunocompromised hosts, organisms are typically abundant, but in healthy patients, they could be more difficult to find. Because the anti-tubercular drug regimen differs between M. tuberculosis and atypical mycobacterial infection, it is especially crucial to differentiate between the two. Rather than the granulomas typical of tuberculosis, MAI frequently exhibits diffuse histiocytic infiltrates and poorly formed granulomas with a high organism count.

The gastrointestinal tract may get infected with other atypical mycobacteria, such as *M. chelonei*, *M. fortuitum*, and *M. sulgai*, which might result in histologic characteristics like those of MAI infection. Molecular tests and culture are useful methods for differentiating between mycobacterial species. The Whipple bacillus is not acid-fast, but MAI is PAS-positive. PCR tests will also be able to differentiate between the two bacteria. A comparable histiocytic infiltrate is produced by Rhodococcus equi, an uncommon infection that is present in immunocompromised people. These intracellular coccobacillary organisms stain with modified acid-fast stains and are both Gram and PAS positive. However, Rhodococcus is more granular on PAS than the MAI bacilli, and it tests negative using a standard Ziehl-Neelsen stain. Molecular tests and culture may also be used to distinguish between these two organisms. Even though MAI stains with both PAS and GMS, fungal species differ morphologically from MAI (Pfaller, 2015).

8.13. Candidiasis

Although it can infect any part of the GI tract, Candida is most commonly seen in esophageal infections. Major abdominal surgery, corticosteroids, chemotherapy, and immunosuppression are common risk factors for invasive Candida infection. The gastrointestinal system serves as a primary entry point for the spread of candidiasis since the infection frequently spreads to ulcers that arise from other sources. It is crucial to distinguish morphologically between superficial colonization and invasive candidiasis since the latter can colonize mucosal surfaces and benign ulcers without invading them. Although *C. tropicalis* and *C. glabrata* may cause similar clinical and pathologic symptoms, *C. albicans* is the most isolated species. It is becoming clear that certain non-albicans species like *Candida krusei* and *Candida parapsilosis* are significant contributors to invasive fungal infections. The esophagus usually has white plaques that show ulcerated mucosa. Candidiasis can present with a variety of macroscopic characteristics, such as ulceration, pseudomembrane development, and inflammatory masses. The colon may appear infarcted if there is a noticeable vascular invasion. Segmental or widespread involvement is possible. Particularly in immunocompromised patients, the corresponding inflammatory response might be mild, exhibiting prominent neutrophilic infiltrates, abscess formation, erosion/ulceration, and necrosis. In the case of pseudomembranes, a blend of fibrin, necrotic debris, and yeast is present. There are also occasionally granulomas. A typical observation in esophageal candidiasis is the presence of many intraepithelial neutrophils in the squamous mucosa of the esophagus, which should prompt the application of fungal stains. Any level of the gut wall can be invaded by fungi, and they can occasionally be clearly seen encroaching on mucosal and submucosal blood vessels. A variety of budding yeast forms, pseudo hyphae, and occasionally real hyphae are produced by *Candida albicans* and *Candida tropicalis* (Negri et al., 2012).

Though it does not develop hyphae or pseudo hyphae, *C. glabrata* has small budding yeast forms that resemble Histoplasma. Other infectious processes are mainly included in the differential diagnosis. Intestinal candidiasis can resemble other inflammatory conditions such as ischemic colitis, pseudomembranous colitis, and chronic idiopathic inflammatory bowel disease. In any immunocompromised patient with ischemic gastrointestinal tract lesions, fungal stains should be carefully considered. It is important to take precautions to prevent mistaking oral Candida infection in the esophagus for actual invasive *Candida esophagitis*. Fungi and associated acute inflammation should be present in the squamous epithelium in cases of invasive candidiasis. Fungi can be observed on the epithelium surface or next to separated squamous cells in cases of oral contamination; there is no accompanying acute inflammation.

8.14. Aspergillosis and Histoplasmosis

Patients with impaired immune systems, especially those experiencing chronic neutropenia, are at risk of developing invasive aspergillus infection of the gastrointestinal tract. As a result, recipients of bone marrow transplants are especially vulnerable to this type of infection. Most aspergillosis patients also have lung abnormalities concurrently. Aspergillus species have replaced the Candida species as the prevalent fungal pathogen. The stomach and esophagus are the common sites of gastrointestinal involvement, after the colon. It is typical to have simultaneous involvement at several sites. While candidiasis is more common in the esophagus, aspergillosis is far less common. A nodular infarction with a zone of ischemic necrosis centered on blood vessels harboring fungi is the typical histologic lesion of aspergillosis. Mucosal lesions with a core necrotic zone with a ring of bleeding may result from these nodular infarctions. Fungal hyphae frequently radiate or grow parallel from the infarct. There is an obvious neutrophilic infiltration and a varied inflammatory response that can range from small to large. Bowel wall transmural infarction is frequently observed. Aspergillus hyphae typically contain septate walls. The lesions generated by Mucor and related zygomycetes are quite similar to those seen in aspergillosis, but intestinal zygomycosis is a rather uncommon condition.

Diabetes and other metabolic acidosis-causing conditions, deferoxamine drugs, other causes of skin and soft tissue disintegration, intravenous drug usage, neonatal prematurity, and malnourishment are all linked to zygomycosis. The symptom is an ulcer, which is frequently big with uneven edges that can resemble cancer. These fungi have the ability to superinfect tissues that have already developed ulcers. Other infectious processes are the main focus of the differential diagnosis, and Aspergillus and zygomycetes can definitely visually mimic each other. Zygomycetes, in contrast to Aspergillus, exhibit broad, irregularly walled, ribbon-like pauciseptate hyphae that randomly branch at different angles.

Fusarium is a filamentous fungal infection that is also linked to neutropenia (Nucci et al., 2021). It is identical to Aspergillus in terms of morphology and closely resembles aspergillosis in terms of clinical and radiographic manifestations. The stomach is not typically affected by ischemia due to atherosclerosis because of its rich blood supply. The Ohio,

Missouri, and Mississippi River basins are home to the endemic *Histoplasma capsulatum* var. *capsulatum*, which is also found in Mexico, Guatemala, Peru, and Venezuela. There have also been reports of histoplasmosis in other non-endemic locations. It is most abundant in soil that has been enhanced by bat or bird droppings. More than 80% of individuals with disseminated infection experience gastrointestinal involvement, and it has a strong preference for spreading through the mononuclear phagocyte system.

BIBLIOGRAPHY

1. Abdel-Salam, O. M. E., Czimmer, J., Debreceni, A., Szolcsányi, J., & Mózsik, G. (2001). Gastric mucosal integrity: Gastric mucosal blood flow and microcirculation. Journal of Physiology-Paris, 95(1), 105–127. https://doi.org/10.1016/S0928-4257(01)00015-8.
2. Abril-Gil, M., Massot-Cladera, M., Pérez-Cano, F. J., Castellote, C., Franch, À., & Castell, M. (2012). A diet enriched with cocoa prevents IgE synthesis in a rat allergy model. Pharmacological Research, 65(6), 603–608. https://doi.org/10.1016/j.phrs.2012.02.001.
3. Allam-Ndoul, B., Guénard, F., Barbier, O., & Vohl, M. C. (2017). A study of the differential effects of eicosapentaenoic acid (EPA) and docosahexaenoic acid (DHA) on gene expression profiles of stimulated THP-1 macrophages. Nutrients, 9(5), 424. https://doi.org/10.3390/nu9050424.
4. Allen, A., & Flemström, G. (2005). Gastroduodenal mucus bicarbonate barrier: Protection against acid and pepsin. American Journal of Physiology–Cell Physiology, 288(1), C1–C19. https://doi.org/10.1152/ajpcell.00102.2004.
5. Amarnath, S., Deeb, L., Philipose, J., Zheng, X., & Gumaste, V. (2021). A comprehensive review of infectious granulomatous diseases of the gastrointestinal tract. Gastroenterology Research and Practice, 2021, 8167149. https://doi.org/10.1155/2021/8167149.
6. Anderson, S. (2017). Acute diarrhoea. In Acute Medicine (pp. 144–149). John Wiley & Sons, Ltd. https://doi.org/10.1002/9781119389613.ch22.
7. Arnold, M., Abnet, C. C., Neale, R. E., Vignat, J., Giovannucci, E. L., McGlynn, K. A., & Bray, F. (2020). Global burden of 5 major types of gastrointestinal cancer. Gastroenterology, 159(1), 335-349.e15. https://doi.org/10.1053/j.gastro.2020.02.068.
8. Babic, T., & Browning, K. N. (2014). The role of vagal neurocircuits in the regulation of nausea and vomiting. European Journal of Pharmacology, 722, 38–47. https://doi.org/10.1016/j.ejphar.2013.08.047.
9. Baker, R. R. (2006). Smoke generation inside a burning cigarette: Modifying combustion to develop cigarettes that may be less hazardous to health. Progress in Energy and Combustion Science, 32(4), 373–385. https://doi.org/10.1016/j.pecs.2006.01.001.

10. Ban, S. (2024). The normal stomach: Anatomy, histology, and specimen dissection relevant to pathological practice. In Morson and Dawson's Gastrointestinal Pathology (pp. 109–127). John Wiley & Sons, Ltd. https://doi.org/10.1002/9781119423195.ch9.
11. Barkun, A., & Leontiadis, G. (2010). Systematic review of the symptom burden, quality of life impairment and costs associated with peptic ulcer disease. The American Journal of Medicine, 123(4), 358–366.e2. https://doi.org/10.1016/j.amjmed.2009.09.031.
12. Bhaijee, F., Arnold, C., Lam-Himlin, D., Montgomery, E. A., & Voltaggio, L. (2015). Infectious mimics of inflammatory bowel disease. Diagnostic Histopathology, 21(7), 267–275. https://doi.org/10.1016/j.mpdhp.2015.06.015.
13. Bhunia, A. K. (2018). Vibrio cholerae, Vibrio parahaemolyticus, and Vibrio vulnificus. In A. K. Bhunia (Ed.), Foodborne Microbial Pathogens: Mechanisms and Pathogenesis (pp. 315–329). New York, NY: Springer. https://doi.org/10.1007/978-1-4939-7349-1_18.
14. Billiauws, L., Maggiori, L., Joly, F., & Panis, Y. (2018). Medical and surgical management of short bowel syndrome. Journal of Visceral Surgery, 155(4), 283–291. https://doi.org/10.1016/j.jviscsurg.2017.12.012.
15. Blum, A. L., Adami, B., Bouzo, M. H., Brandstätter, G., Fumagalli, I., Galmiche, J. P., & The Italian Eurocis Trialists. (1993). Effect of cisapride on relapse of esophagitis. Digestive Diseases and Sciences, 38(3), 551–560. https://doi.org/10.1007/BF01316514.
16. Boparai, V., Rajagopalan, J., & Triadafilopoulos, G. (2008). Guide to the use of proton pump inhibitors in adult patients. Drugs, 68(7), 925–947. https://doi.org/10.2165/00003495-200868070-00004.
17. Borrelli, F., Capasso, R., Russo, A., & Ernst, E. (2004). Green tea and gastrointestinal cancer risk. Alimentary Pharmacology & Therapeutics, 19(5), 497–510. https://doi.org/10.1111/j.1365-2036.2004.01884.x.
18. Bossi, P., Delrio, P., Mascheroni, A., & Zanetti, M. (2021). The spectrum of malnutrition/cachexia/sarcopenia in oncology according to different cancer types and settings: A narrative review. Nutrients, 13(6), 1980. https://doi.org/10.3390/nu13061980.
19. Briassoulis, G. (2014). Nutrition monitoring in the PICU. In D. S. Wheeler, H. R. Wong, & T. P. Shanley (Eds.), Pediatric Critical Care Medicine: Volume 1: Care of the Critically Ill or Injured Child (pp. 579–601). London: Springer. https://doi.org/10.1007/978-1-4471-6362-6_42.
20. Brown, S. R., & Adam, I. (2002). Intestinal obstruction. Surgery (Oxford), 20(7), 157–164. https://doi.org/10.1383/surg.20.7.157.14394.
21. Businello, G., Dal Pozzo, C. A., Sbaraglia, M., Mastracci, L., Milione, M., Saragoni, L., & Fassan, M. (2020). Histopathological landscape of rare oesophageal neoplasms. World Journal of Gastroenterology, 26(27), 3865–3888. https://doi.org/10.3748/wjg.v26.i27.3865.
22. Calder, P. C. (2001). Polyunsaturated fatty acids, inflammation, and immunity. Lipids, 36(9), 1007–1024. https://doi.org/10.1007/s11745-001-0812-7.
23. Camilleri, M., Malhi, H., & Acosta, A. (2017). Gastrointestinal complications of obesity. Gastroenterology, 152(7), 1656–1670. https://doi.org/10.1053/j.gastro.2016.12.052.
24. Camps-Bossacoma, M., Pérez-Cano, F. J., Franch, À., Untersmayr, E., & Castell, M. (2017). Effect of a cocoa diet on the small intestine and gut-associated lymphoid tissue composition in an oral sensitization model in rats. The Journal of Nutritional Biochemistry, 42, 182–193. https://doi.org/10.1016/j.jnutbio.2017.01.005.

25. Chan, F. K., & Leung, W. K. (2002). Peptic-ulcer disease. The Lancet, 360(9337), 933–941. https://doi.org/10.1016/S0140-6736(02)11030-0.

26. Chou, C. L., Lin, J. K., Wang, H. S., Yang, S. H., Li, A. F. Y., & Chang, S. C. (2010). Microsatellite instability screening should be done for right-sided colon cancer patients less than 60 years of age. International Journal of Colorectal Disease, 25(1), 47–52. https://doi.org/10.1007/s00384-009-0815-y.

27. Corfield, A. P. (2015). Mucins: A biologically relevant glycan barrier in mucosal protection. Biochimica et Biophysica Acta (BBA)–General Subjects, 1850(1), 236–252. https://doi.org/10.1016/j.bbagen.2014.05.003.

28. Costa, M., & Furness, J. B. (1982). Nervous control of intestinal motility. In G. Bertaccini (Ed.), Mediators and Drugs in Gastrointestinal Motility I: Morphological Basis and Neurophysiological Control (pp. 279–382). Berlin, Heidelberg: Springer. https://doi.org/10.1007/978-3-642-68437-1_10.

29. Crabtree, J. (1996). Gastric mucosal inflammatory responses to Helicobacter pylori. Alimentary Pharmacology & Therapeutics, 10(Sup1), 29–37. https://doi.org/10.1046/j.1365-2036.1996.22164003.x.

30. Cuomo-Granston, A., & Drummond, P. D. (2010). Migraine and motion sickness: What is the link? Progress in Neurobiology, 91(4), 300–312. https://doi.org/10.1016/j.pneurobio.2010.04.001.

31. Daniels, I. R., & Allum, W. H. (2005). The anatomy and physiology of the stomach. In J. W. L. Fielding & M. T. Hallissey (Eds.), Upper Gastrointestinal Surgery (pp. 17–37). London: Springer. https://doi.org/10.1007/1-84628-066-4_2.

32. Davani-Davari, D., Negahdaripour, M., Karimzadeh, I., Seifan, M., Mohkam, M., Masoumi, S. J., & Ghasemi, Y. (2019). Prebiotics: Definition, types, sources, mechanisms, and clinical applications. Foods, 8(3), 92. https://doi.org/10.3390/foods8030092.

33. Davis, M. P., & Walsh, D. (2000). Treatment of nausea and vomiting in advanced cancer. Supportive Care in Cancer, 8(6), 444–452. https://doi.org/10.1007/s005200000151.

34. De Fazio, L., Beghetti, I., Bertuccio, S. N., Marsico, C., Martini, S., Masetti, R., & Aceti, A. (2021). Necrotizing enterocolitis: Overview on in vitro models. International Journal of Molecular Sciences, 22(13), 6761. https://doi.org/10.3390/ijms22136761.

35. Di Saverio, S., Bassi, M., Smerieri, N., Masetti, M., Ferrara, F., Fabbri, C., & Jovine, E. (2014). Diagnosis and treatment of perforated or bleeding peptic ulcers: 2013 WSES position paper. World Journal of Emergency Surgery, 9(1), 45. https://doi.org/10.1186/1749-7922-9-45.

36. Dilli, D., Eras, Z., Özkan Ulu, H., Dilmen, U., & Durgut Şakrucu, E. (2012). Does necrotizing enterocolitis affect growth and neurodevelopmental outcome in very low birth weight infants? Pediatric Surgery International, 28(5), 471–476. https://doi.org/10.1007/s00383-012-3051-4.

37. Disca, V., Capuano, E., & Arlorio, M. (2024). Colonic fermentation of enzymatically treated cocoa bean shells (CBSs) and short chain fatty acids (SCFAs) production. LWT, 202, 116311. https://doi.org/10.1016/j.lwt.2024.116311.

38. Doroftei, B., Ilie, O. D., Armeanu, T., Stoian, I. L., Anton, N., Babici, R. G., & Ilea, C. (2023). A narrative review discussing the obstetric repercussions due to alterations of personalized bacterial sites developed within the vagina, cervix, and endometrium. Journal of Clinical Medicine, 12(15), 5069. https://doi.org/10.3390/jcm12155069.

39. DuPont, H. L., Jiang, Z. D., Alexander, A. S., DuPont, A. W., & Brown, E. L. (2023). Intestinal IgA-coated bacteria in healthy- and altered-microbiomes (dysbiosis) and predictive value in successful fecal microbiota transplantation. Microorganisms, 11(1), 93. https://doi.org/10.3390/microorganisms11010093.

40. Elstner, E. F. (1987). 8—Metabolism of activated oxygen species. In D. D. Davies (Ed.), Biochemistry of Metabolism (pp. 253–315). Academic Press. https://doi.org/10.1016/B978-0-12-675411-7.50014-8.

41. Er, T. K., Chen, C. C., Bujanda, L., & Herreros-Villanueva, M. (2014). Clinical relevance of KRAS mutations in codon 13: Where are we? Cancer Letters, 343(1), 1–5. https://doi.org/10.1016/j.canlet.2013.09.012.

42. Ergenekon, E., Tayman, C., & Özkan, H. (2021). Turkish Neonatal Society necrotizing enterocolitis diagnosis, treatment and prevention guidelines. Turkish Archives of Pediatrics, 56(5), 513–524. https://doi.org/10.5152/TurkArchPediatr.2021.21164.

43. Fanning, S., Hall, L. J., & van Sinderen, D. (2012). Bifidobacterium breve UCC2003 surface exopolysaccharide production is a beneficial trait mediating commensal-host interaction through immune modulation and pathogen protection. Gut Microbes, 3(5), 420–425. https://doi.org/10.4161/gmic.20630.

44. Farmer, A. D., Gallagher, J., Bruckner-Holt, C., & Aziz, Q. (2017). Narcotic bowel syndrome. The Lancet Gastroenterology & Hepatology, 2(5), 361–368. https://doi.org/10.1016/S2468-1253(16)30217-5.

45. Farnebo, M., Bykov, V. J. N., & Wiman, K. G. (2010). The p53 tumor suppressor: A master regulator of diverse cellular processes and therapeutic target in cancer. Biochemical and Biophysical Research Communications, 396(1), 85–89. https://doi.org/10.1016/j.bbrc.2010.02.152.

46. Ferreira, T. M., Leonel, A. J., Melo, M. A., Santos, R. R. G., Cara, D. C., Cardoso, V. N., & Alvarez-Leite, J. I. (2012). Oral supplementation of butyrate reduces mucositis and intestinal permeability associated with 5-fluorouracil administration. Lipids, 47(7), 669–678. https://doi.org/10.1007/s11745-012-3680-3.

47. Festen, H. P. M. (1991). Intrinsic factor secretion and cobalamin absorption: Physiology and pathophysiology in the gastrointestinal tract. Scandinavian Journal of Gastroenterology, 26(sup188), 1–7. https://doi.org/10.3109/00365529109111222.

48. Fijan, S. (2014). Microorganisms with claimed probiotic properties: An overview of recent literature. International Journal of Environmental Research and Public Health, 11(5), 4745–4767. https://doi.org/10.3390/ijerph110504745.

49. Freitas, M., Gomes, A., Porto, G., & Fernandes, E. (2010). Nickel induces oxidative burst, NF-κB activation and interleukin-8 production in human neutrophils. JBIC Journal of Biological Inorganic Chemistry, 15(8), 1275–1283. https://doi.org/10.1007/s00775-010-0685-3.

50. Galindo, C. L., Rosenzweig, J. A., Kirtley, M. L., & Chopra, A. K. (2011). Pathogenesis of Yersinia enterocolitica and Yersinia pseudotuberculosis in human yersiniosis. Journal of Pathogens, 2011, 182051. https://doi.org/10.4061/2011/182051.

51. Gascon, J., Vila, J., Valls, M. E., Ruiz, L., Vidal, J., Corachan, M., & De Anta Jimenez, M. T. (1993). Etiology of traveller's diarrhea in Spanish travellers to developing countries. European Journal of Epidemiology, 9(2), 217–223. https://doi.org/10.1007/BF00158796.

52. Gisbert, J. P., Niño, P., Cara, C., & Rodrigo, L. (2008). Comparative effectiveness of azathioprine in Crohn's disease and ulcerative colitis: Prospective, long-term, follow-up study of 394 patients. Alimentary Pharmacology & Therapeutics, 28(2), 228–238. https://doi.org/10.1111/j.1365-2036.2008.03732.x.

53. Gisondi, P., Fantuzzi, F., Malerba, M., & Girolomoni, G. (2007). Folic acid in general medicine and dermatology. Journal of Dermatological Treatment, 18(3), 138–146. https://doi.org/10.1080/09546630701247930.

54. Goulart, R. de A., Barbalho, S. M., Gasparini, R. G., & de Carvalho, A. de C. A. (2016). Facing terminal ileitis: Going beyond Crohn's disease. Gastroenterology Research, 9(1), 1–9. https://doi.org/10.14740/gr698w.

55. Graham, D. Y., Lu, H., & Yamaoka, Y. (2008). Therapy for Helicobacter pylori infection can be improved. Drugs, 68(6), 725–736. https://doi.org/10.2165/00003495-200868060-00001.

56. Gridelli, C., Rossi, A., Carbone, D. P., Guarize, J., Karachaliou, N., Mok, T., & Rosell, R. (2015). Non-small-cell lung cancer. Nature Reviews Disease Primers, 1(1), 1–16. https://doi.org/10.1038/nrdp.2015.9.

57. Hanna, G. B., Shimi, S. M., & Cuschieri, S. A. (2014). Disorders of the oesophagus. In Essential Surgical Practice (5th ed.). CRC Press.

58. Iijima, S. (2024). Clinical dilemma involving treatments for very low-birth-weight infants and the potential risk of necrotizing enterocolitis: A narrative literature review. Journal of Clinical Medicine, 13(1), 62. https://doi.org/10.3390/jcm13010062.

59. Inchingolo, F., Inchingolo, A. M., Latini, G., Ferrante, L., de Ruvo, E., Campanelli, M., & Dipalma, G. (2024). Difference in the intestinal microbiota between breastfed infants and infants fed with artificial milk: A systematic review. Pathogens, 13(7), 533. https://doi.org/10.3390/pathogens13070533.

60. Jasielska, M., & Grzybowska-Chlebowczyk, U. (2021). Hypocalcemia and vitamin D deficiency in children with inflammatory bowel diseases and lactose intolerance. Nutrients, 13(8), 2583. https://doi.org/10.3390/nu13082583.

61. Javelli, D. R. (2015). Diet and nutrition in the treatment of Crohn's disease. In A. Fichera & M. K. Krane (Eds.), Crohn's Disease: Basic Principles (pp. 265–279). Cham: Springer International Publishing. https://doi.org/10.1007/978-3-319-14181-7_21.

62. Joosten, E., Vanderelst, B., & Pelemans, W. (1999). The effect of different diagnostic criteria on the prevalence of malnutrition in a hospitalized geriatric population. Aging Clinical and Experimental Research, 11(6), 390–394. https://doi.org/10.1007/BF03339818.

63. Kaneko, H., Konagaya, T., & Kusugami, K. (2002). Helicobacter pylori and gut hormones. Journal of Gastroenterology, 37(2), 77–86. https://doi.org/10.1007/s005350200000.

64. Kerr, J., Anderson, C., & Lippman, S. M. (2017). Physical activity, sedentary behaviour, diet, and cancer: An update and emerging new evidence. The Lancet Oncology, 18(8), e457–e471. https://doi.org/10.1016/S1470-2045(17)30411-4.

65. Khan, F. Y., Kamha, A. A., & Alomary, I. Y. (2006). Fulminant hepatic failure caused by Salmonella paratyphi A infection. World Journal of Gastroenterology: WJG, 12(32), 5253–5255. https://doi.org/10.3748/wjg.v12.i32.5253.

66. Khan, S., Andrews, K. L., & Chin-Dusting, J. P. F. (2019). Cyclo-oxygenase (COX) inhibitors and cardiovascular risk: Are non-steroidal anti-inflammatory drugs really anti-inflammatory? International Journal of Molecular Sciences, 20(17), 4262. https://doi.org/10.3390/ijms20174262.

67. Kim, H. P., Crockett, S. D., & Shaheen, N. J. (2014). The burden of gastrointestinal and liver disease around the world. In GI Epidemiology (pp. 1–13). John Wiley & Sons, Ltd. https://doi.org/10.1002/9781118727072.ch1.

68. Koort, K., Sõsa, K., Türk, S., Lapp, E., Talving, E., Karits, P., & Mändar, R. (2023). Lactobacillus crispatus-dominated vaginal microbiome and Acinetobacter-dominated seminal microbiome support beneficial ART outcome. Acta Obstetricia et Gynecologica Scandinavica, 102(7), 921–934. https://doi.org/10.1111/aogs.14598.

69. Laillou, A., Pfanner, S., Chan, T., Chea, C., Mam, B., Sambath, P., & Wieringa, F. (2016). Beyond effectiveness—The adversities of implementing a fortification program. A case study on the quality of iron fortification of fish and soy sauce in Cambodia. Nutrients, 8(2), 94. https://doi.org/10.3390/nu8020094.

70. Lamps, L. W. (2010). Helicobacter pylori and related species. In L. W. Lamps (Ed.), Surgical Pathology of the Gastrointestinal System: Bacterial, Fungal, Viral, and Parasitic Infections (pp. 17–26). New York, NY: Springer US. https://doi.org/10.1007/978-1-4419-0861-2_4.

71. Lee, J. K. F., Hern Tan, L. T., Ramadas, A., Ab Mutalib, N. S., & Lee, L. H. (2020). Exploring the role of gut bacteria in health and disease in preterm neonates. International Journal of Environmental Research and Public Health, 17(19), 6963. https://doi.org/10.3390/ijerph17196963.

72. Leu, S. B., Shulman, S. C., Steelman, C. K., Lamps, L. W., Bulut, O. P., Abramowsky, C. R., & Shehata, B. M. (2013). Pathogenic Yersinia DNA in intestinal specimens of pediatric patients with Crohn's disease. Fetal and Pediatric Pathology, 32(5), 367–370. https://doi.org/10.3109/15513815.2013.768744.

73. Li, S., Gao, Y., Shang, Q., Guo, W., Liu, H., Wei, J., & Chen, T. (2021). Evidence for the existence of microbiota in the placenta and blood of pregnant mice exposed to various bacteria. Medicine in Microecology, 8, 100040. https://doi.org/10.1016/j.medmic.2021.100040.

74. Lindkvist, B., Johansen, D., Stocks, T., Concin, H., Bjørge, T., Almquist, M., & Manjer, J. (2014). Metabolic risk factors for esophageal squamous cell carcinoma and adenocarcinoma: A prospective study of 580,000 subjects within the Me-Can project. BMC Cancer, 14(1), 103. https://doi.org/10.1186/1471-2407-14-103.

75. Liszt, K. I., Ley, J. P., Lieder, B., Behrens, M., Stöger, V., Reiner, A., & Somoza, V. (2017). Caffeine induces gastric acid secretion via bitter taste signaling in gastric parietal cells. Proceedings of the National Academy of Sciences, 114(30), E6260–E6269. https://doi.org/10.1073/pnas.1703728114.

76. Locke, G. R., Talley, N. J., Fett, S. L., Zinsmeister, A. R., & Melton, L. J. (1999). Risk factors associated with symptoms of gastroesophageal reflux. The American Journal of Medicine, 106(6), 642–649. https://doi.org/10.1016/S0002-9343(99)00121-7.

77. Lu, C. L., Chang, S. S., Wang, S. S., Chang, F. Y., & Lee, S. D. (2004). Silent peptic ulcer disease: Frequency, factors leading to "silence," and implications regarding the pathogenesis of visceral symptoms. Gastrointestinal Endoscopy, 60(1), 34–38. https://doi.org/10.1016/S0016-5107(04)01311-2.

78. Malumbres, M. (2014). Cyclin-dependent kinases. Genome Biology, 15(6), 122. https://doi.org/10.1186/gb4184.

79. Marć, M. A., Jastrząb, R., & Mytych, J. (2022). Does the gut microbial metabolome really matter? The connection between gut metabolome and neurological disorders. Nutrients, 14(19), 3967. https://doi.org/10.3390/nu14193967.

80. Massironi, S., Cavalcoli, F., Rausa, E., Invernizzi, P., Braga, M., & Vecchi, M. (2020). Understanding short bowel syndrome: Current status and future perspectives. Digestive and Liver Disease, 52(3), 253–261. https://doi.org/10.1016/j.dld.2019.11.013.

81. Matarese, L. E., O'Keefe, S. J., Kandil, H. M., Bond, G., Costa, G., & Abu-Elmagd, K. (2005). Short bowel syndrome: Clinical guidelines for nutrition management. Nutrition in Clinical Practice, 20(5), 493–502. https://doi.org/10.1177/0115426505020005493.

82. McCubrey, J. A., Steelman, L. S., Chappell, W. H., Abrams, S. L., Montalto, G., Cervello, M., & Martelli, A. M. (2012). Mutations and deregulation of Ras/Raf/MEK/ERK and PI3K/PTEN/Akt/mTOR cascades which alter therapy response. Oncotarget, 3(9), 954–987. https://www.ncbi.nlm.nih.gov/pmc/articles/PMC3660063/ (accessed on 21 October 2024).

83. McFarland, L. V. (2021). Efficacy of single-strain probiotics versus multi-strain mixtures: Systematic review of strain and disease specificity. Digestive Diseases and Sciences, 66(3), 694–704. https://doi.org/10.1007/s10620-020-06244-z.

84. Mercer, E. M., & Arrieta, M. C. (2023). Probiotics to improve the gut microbiome in premature infants: Are we there yet? Gut Microbes, 15(1), 2201160. https://doi.org/10.1080/19490976.2023.2201160.

85. Miller, T. E., Raghunathan, K., & Gan, T. J. (2014). State-of-the-art fluid management in the operating room. Best Practice & Research Clinical Anaesthesiology, 28(3), 261–273. https://doi.org/10.1016/j.bpa.2014.07.003.

86. Montoro-Huguet, M. A., Belloc, B., & Domínguez-Cajal, M. (2021). Small and large intestine (I): Malabsorption of nutrients. Nutrients, 13(4), 1254. https://doi.org/10.3390/nu13041254.

87. Morita, I. (2002). Distinct functions of COX-1 and COX-2. Prostaglandins & Other Lipid Mediators, 68, 69, 165–175. https://doi.org/10.1016/S0090-6980(02)00029-1.

88. Moyer, N. P. (1987). Clinical significance of Aeromonas species isolated from patients with diarrhea. Journal of Clinical Microbiology, 25(11), 2044–2048. https://doi.org/10.1128/jcm.25.11.2044-2048.1987.

89. Nair, J. R., & Moots, R. J. (2017). Behcet's disease. Clinical Medicine, 17(1), 71–77. https://doi.org/10.7861/clinmedicine.17-1-71.

90. Negri, M., Silva, S., Henriques, M., & Oliveira, R. (2012). Insights into Candida tropicalis nosocomial infections and virulence factors. European Journal of Clinical Microbiology & Infectious Diseases, 31(7), 1399–1412. https://doi.org/10.1007/s10096-011-1455-z.

91. Nucci, M., Barreiros, G., Akiti, T., Anaissie, E., & Nouér, S. A. (2021). Invasive fusariosis in patients with hematologic diseases. Journal of Fungi, 7(10), 815. https://doi.org/10.3390/jof7100815.

92. Oh, N. S., Lee, J. Y., Kim, Y. T., Kim, S. H., & Lee, J. H. (2020). Cancer-protective effect of a synbiotic combination between Lactobacillus gasseri 505 and a Cudrania tricuspidata leaf

extract on colitis-associated colorectal cancer. Gut Microbes, 12(1), 1785803. https://doi.org/10.1080/19490976.2020.1785803.

93. Okburan, G., & Kızıler, S. (2023). Human milk oligosaccharides as prebiotics. Pediatrics & Neonatology, 64(3), 231–238. https://doi.org/10.1016/j.pedneo.2022.09.017.

94. Ortiz, M. del C., Lores-Arnaiz, S., Albertoni Borghese, M. F., Balonga, S., Lavagna, A., Filipuzzi, A. L., & Bustamante, J. (2013). Mitochondrial dysfunction in brain cortex mitochondria of STZ-diabetic rats: Effect of l-arginine. Neurochemical Research, 38(12), 2570–2580. https://doi.org/10.1007/s11064-013-1172-3.

95. Oshima, T., & Miwa, H. (2016). Gastrointestinal mucosal barrier function and diseases. Journal of Gastroenterology, 51(8), 768–778. https://doi.org/10.1007/s00535-016-1207-z.

96. Otuya, D. O., Verma, Y., Farrokhi, H., Higgins, L., Rosenberg, M., Damman, C., & Tearney, G. J. (2018). Non-endoscopic biopsy techniques: A review. Expert Review of Gastroenterology & Hepatology, 12(2), 109–117. https://doi.org/10.1080/17474124.2018.1412828.

97. Pandey, K. R., Naik, S. R., & Vakil, B. V. (2015). Probiotics, prebiotics and synbiotics: A review. Journal of Food Science and Technology, 52(12), 7577–7587. https://doi.org/10.1007/s13197-015-1921-1.

98. Parkin, K., Christophersen, C. T., Verhasselt, V., Cooper, M. N., & Martino, D. (2021). Risk factors for gut dysbiosis in early life. Microorganisms, 9(10), 2066. https://doi.org/10.3390/microorganisms9102066.

99. Parronchi, P., Romagnani, P., Annunziato, F., Sampognaro, S., Becchio, A., Giannarini, L., & Romagnani, S. (1997). Type 1 T-helper cell predominance and interleukin-12 expression in the gut of patients with Crohn's disease. The American Journal of Pathology, 150(3), 823–832. https://www.ncbi.nlm.nih.gov/pmc/articles/PMC1857889/ (accessed on 21 October 2024).

100. Peek, S. F., McGuirk, S. M., Sweeney, R. W., & Cummings, K. J. (2018). Infectious diseases of the gastrointestinal tract. In Rebhun's Diseases of Dairy Cattle (pp. 249–356). https://doi.org/10.1016/B978-0-323-39055-2.00006-1.

101. Periti, P., Tonelli, F., Capurso, L., & Nicoletti, P. (1999). Managing Helicobacter pylori infection in the new millennium: A review. Journal of Chemotherapy, 11(sup4), 3–55. https://doi.org/10.1080/1120009X.1999.11782276.

102. Peura, D. A. (2004). Prevention of nonsteroidal anti-inflammatory drug-associated gastrointestinal symptoms and ulcer complications. The American Journal of Medicine Supplements, 117(5, Supplement 1), 63–71. https://doi.org/10.1016/j.amjmed.2004.07.010.

103. Pfaller, M. A. (2015). Chapter 7—Invasive fungal infections and approaches to their diagnosis. In A. Sails & Y. W. Tang (Eds.), Methods in Microbiology (pp. 219–287). Academic Press. https://doi.org/10.1016/bs.mim.2015.05.002.

104. Pflughoeft, K. J., & Versalovic, J. (2012). Human microbiome in health and disease. Annual Review of Pathology: Mechanisms of Disease, 7, 99–122. https://doi.org/10.1146/annurev-pathol-011811-132421.

105. Piechota-Polanczyk, A., & Fichna, J. (2014). The role of oxidative stress in pathogenesis and treatment of inflammatory bowel diseases. Naunyn-Schmiedeberg's Archives of Pharmacology, 387(7), 605–620. https://doi.org/10.1007/s00210-014-0985-1.

106. Pirlich, M., & Lochs, H. (2001). Nutrition in the elderly. Best Practice & Research Clinical

Gastroenterology, 15(6), 869–884. https://doi.org/10.1053/bega.2001.0246.

107. Poehlmann, A., Kuester, D., Malfertheiner, P., Guenther, T., & Roessner, A. (2012). Inflammation and Barrett's carcinogenesis. Pathology–Research and Practice, 208(5), 269–280. https://doi.org/10.1016/j.prp.2012.03.007.

108. Qiao, Y., Zhang, K., Zhang, Z., Zhang, C., Sun, Y., & Feng, Z. (2022). Fermented soybean foods: A review of their functional components, mechanism of action and factors influencing their health benefits. Food Research International, 158, 111575. https://doi.org/10.1016/j.foodres.2022.111575.

109. Quigley, E. M. M. (2017). Prokinetics in the management of functional gastrointestinal disorders. Current Gastroenterology Reports, 19(10), 53. https://doi.org/10.1007/s11894-017-0593-6.

110. Rasheed, S., Zinicola, R., Watson, D., Bajwa, A., & McDonald, P. J. (2007). Intra-abdominal and gastrointestinal tuberculosis. Colorectal Disease, 9(9), 773–783. https://doi.org/10.1111/j.1463-1318.2007.01337.x.

111. Reinhardt, G. F., Myscofski, J. W., Wilkens, D. B., Dobrin, P. B., Mangan, J. R., & Stannard, R. T. (1980). Incidence and mortality of hypoalbuminemic patients in hospitalized veterans. Journal of Parenteral and Enteral Nutrition, 4(4), 357–359. https://doi.org/10.1177/014860718000400404.

112. Ribeiro, R. A., Wanderley, C. W. S., Wong, D. V. T., Mota, J. M. S. C., Leite, C. A. V. G., Souza, M. H. L. P., & Lima-Júnior, R. C. P. (2016). Irinotecan- and 5-fluorouracil-induced intestinal mucositis: Insights into pathogenesis and therapeutic perspectives. Cancer Chemotherapy and Pharmacology, 78(5), 881–893. https://doi.org/10.1007/s00280-016-3139-y.

113. Rinninella, E., Raoul, P., Cintoni, M., Franceschi, F., Miggiano, G. A. D., Gasbarrini, A., & Mele, M. C. (2019). What is the healthy gut microbiota composition? A changing ecosystem across age, environment, diet, and diseases. Microorganisms, 7(1), 14. https://doi.org/10.3390/microorganisms7010014.

114. Rojo-Poveda, O., Barbosa-Pereira, L., Zeppa, G., & Stévigny, C. (2020). Cocoa bean shell—a by-product with nutritional properties and biofunctional potential. Nutrients, 12(4), 1123. https://doi.org/10.3390/nu12041123.

115. Saadaoui, M., Singh, P., & Al Khodor, S. (2021). Oral microbiome and pregnancy: A bidirectional relationship. Journal of Reproductive Immunology, 145, 103293. https://doi.org/10.1016/j.jri.2021.103293.

116. Sachs, G. (1997). Proton pump inhibitors and acid-related diseases. Pharmacotherapy: The Journal of Human Pharmacology and Drug Therapy, 17(1), 22–37. https://doi.org/10.1002/j.1875-9114.1997.tb03675.x.

117. Schneider, A., & Whitcomb, D. C. (2002). Hereditary pancreatitis: A model for inflammatory diseases of the pancreas. Best Practice & Research Clinical Gastroenterology, 16(3), 347–363. https://doi.org/10.1053/bega.2002.0311.

118. Seddighi, R., & Lee, L. (2016). Complications associated with nonsteroidal anti-inflammatory drugs. In Complications in Small Animal Surgery (pp. 97–109). John Wiley & Sons, Ltd. https://doi.org/10.1002/9781119421344.ch15.

119. Seki, H., Tani, Y., & Arita, M. (2009). Omega-3 PUFA derived anti-inflammatory lipid mediator resolvin E1. Prostaglandins & Other Lipid Mediators, 89(3), 126–130. https://doi.org/10.1016/j.prostaglandins.2009.03.002.

120. Seo, S. H., Kim, S. E., Kang, Y. K., Ryoo, B. Y., Ryu, M. H., Jeong, J. H., & Sung, M. K. (2016). Association of nutritional status-related indices and chemotherapy-induced adverse events in gastric cancer patients. BMC Cancer, 16(1), 900. https://doi.org/10.1186/s12885-016-2934-5.

121. Sergi, C. M. (2020). Gastrointestinal tract. In Pathology of Childhood and Adolescence: An Illustrated Guide (pp. 255–424). Springer. https://doi.org/10.1007/978-3-662-59169-7_3.

122. Shapiro, A. C., Wu, D., Hayek, M. G., Meydani, M., & Meydani, S. N. (1994). Role of eicosanoids and vitamin E in fish oil-induced changes of splenocyte proliferation to T cell mitogens in mice. Nutrition Research, 14(9), 1339–1354. https://doi.org/10.1016/S0271-5317(05)80294-5.

123. Sheppe, A. E. F., & Edelmann, M. J. (2021). Roles of eicosanoids in regulating inflammation and neutrophil migration as an innate host response to bacterial infections. Infection and Immunity, 89(8). https://doi.org/10.1128/iai.00095-21.

124. Sjöblom, M. (2005). The duodenal mucosal bicarbonate secretion. Upsala Journal of Medical Sciences, 110(2), 115–150. https://doi.org/10.3109/2000-1967-076.

125. Soares, T. F., & Oliveira, M. B. P. P. (2022). Cocoa by-products: Characterization of bioactive compounds and beneficial health effects. Molecules, 27(5), 1625. https://doi.org/10.3390/molecules27051625.

126. Sohn, E. J., Goralsky, J. A., Shay, J. W., & Min, J. (2023). The molecular mechanisms and therapeutic prospects of alternative lengthening of telomeres (ALT). Cancers, 15(7), 1945. https://doi.org/10.3390/cancers15071945.

127. Sorrenti, V., Ali, S., Mancin, L., Davinelli, S., Paoli, A., & Scapagnini, G. (2020). Cocoa polyphenols and gut microbiota interplay: Bioavailability, prebiotic effect, and impact on human health. Nutrients, 12(7), 1908. https://doi.org/10.3390/nu12071908.

128. Sousa, S., Lecuit, M., & Cossart, P. (2005). Microbial strategies to target, cross or disrupt epithelia. Current Opinion in Cell Biology, 17(5), 489–498. https://doi.org/10.1016/j.ceb.2005.08.013.

129. Spahn, T. W., Weiner, H. L., Rennert, P. D., Lügering, N., Fontana, A., Domschke, W., & Kucharzik, T. (2002). Mesenteric lymph nodes are critical for the induction of high-dose oral tolerance in the absence of Peyer's patches. European Journal of Immunology, 32(4), 1109–1113. https://doi.org/10.1002/1521-4141(200204)32:4<1109::AID-IMMU1109>3.0.CO;2-K.

130. Spainhour, C. B. (2018). Gastrointestinal function and toxicology in canines. In Toxicology of the Gastrointestinal Tract (2nd ed.). CRC Press.

131. Steckel, R. H. (2024). Anthropometrics. In C. Diebolt & M. Haupert (Eds.), Handbook of Cliometrics (pp. 1787–1805). Springer International Publishing. https://doi.org/10.1007/978-3-031-35583-7_61.

132. Tack, J., & Pandolfino, J. E. (2018). Pathophysiology of gastroesophageal reflux disease. Gastroenterology, 154(2), 277–288. https://doi.org/10.1053/j.gastro.2017.09.047.

133. Taherali, F., Varum, F., & Basit, A. W. (2018). A slippery slope: On the origin, role and physiology of mucus. Advanced Drug Delivery Reviews, 124, 16–33. https://doi.org/10.1016/j.addr.2017.10.014.

134. Tsuchida, N., Murugan, A. K., & Grieco, M. (2016). Kirsten Ras oncogene: Significance of its discovery in human cancer research. Oncotarget, 7(29), 46717–46733. https://doi.org/10.18632/oncotarget.8773.

135. Tunis, S. R., Sheinhait, I. A., Schmid, C. H., Bishop, D. J., & Ross, S. D. (1997). Lansoprazole compared with histamine2-receptor antagonists in healing gastric ulcers: A meta-analysis. Clinical Therapeutics, 19(4), 743–757. https://doi.org/10.1016/S0149-2918(97)80098-7.

136. Unge, P. (1999). Antibiotic treatment of Helicobacter pylori infection. In T. U. Westblom, S. J. Czinn, & J. G. Nedrud (Eds.), Gastroduodenal Disease and Helicobacter pylori: Pathophysiology, Diagnosis and Treatment (pp. 261–300). Springer. https://doi.org/10.1007/978-3-642-60013-5_13.

137. Van Cutsem, E., & Arends, J. (2005). The causes and consequences of cancer-associated malnutrition. European Journal of Oncology Nursing, 9, S51–S63. https://doi.org/10.1016/j.ejon.2005.09.007.

138. Van Gossum, A., Cabre, E., Hébuterne, X., Jeppesen, P., Krznaric, Z., Messing, B., & Nightingale, J. (2009). ESPEN guidelines on parenteral nutrition: Gastroenterology. Clinical Nutrition, 28(4), 415–427. https://doi.org/10.1016/j.clnu.2009.04.022.

139. Vasina, V., Broccoli, M., Ursino, M. G., Bellot, S. F., Soleti, A., Paolini, M., & De Ponti, F. (2009). Effects of the non-peptidyl low molecular weight radical scavenger IAC in DNBS-induced colitis in rats. European Journal of Pharmacology, 614(1), 137–145. https://doi.org/10.1016/j.ejphar.2009.04.021.

140. Venerito, M., & Malfertheiner, P. (2010). Interaction of Helicobacter pylori infection and nonsteroidal anti-inflammatory drugs in gastric and duodenal ulcers. Helicobacter, 15(4), 239–250. https://doi.org/10.1111/j.1523-5378.2010.00762.x.

141. Vinderola, G., Sanders, M. E., & Salminen, S. (2022). The concept of postbiotics. Foods, 11(8), 1077. https://doi.org/10.3390/foods11081077.

142. Vives-Bauza, C., Starkov, A., & Garcia-Arumi, E. (2007). Measurements of the antioxidant enzyme activities of superoxide dismutase, catalase, and glutathione peroxidase. In Mitochondria (2nd ed., Vol. 80, pp. 379–393). Academic Press. https://doi.org/10.1016/S0091-679X(06)80019-1.

143. Wahlqvist, M. L., & Wattanapenpaiboon, N. (2020). Food digestion. In Food and Nutrition (4th ed.). Routledge.

144. Wan, L. Y. M., Chen, Z. J., Shah, N. P., & El-Nezami, H. (2016). Modulation of intestinal epithelial defense responses by probiotic bacteria. Critical Reviews in Food Science and Nutrition, 56(16), 2628–2641. https://doi.org/10.1080/10408398.2014.905450.

145. Washington, N., & Wilson, C. G. (1986). Antacids: Physiology versus pharmaceutics. International Journal of Pharmaceutics, 28(2), 249–260. https://doi.org/10.1016/0378-5173(86)90251-6.

146. Wee, P., & Wang, Z. (2017). Epidermal growth factor receptor cell proliferation signaling pathways. Cancers, 9(5), 52. https://doi.org/10.3390/cancers9050052.

147. Xu, X. Y., Meng, X., Li, S., Gan, R. Y., Li, Y., & Li, H. B. (2018). Bioactivity, health benefits, and related molecular mechanisms of curcumin: Current progress, challenges, and perspectives. Nutrients, 10(10), 1553. https://doi.org/10.3390/nu10101553.

148. Yaghoobi, M., & Armstrong, D. (2022). Peptic ulcer disease. In Yamada's Textbook of Gastroenterology (pp. 924–976). John Wiley & Sons, Ltd. https://doi.org/10.1002/9781119600206.ch49.

149. Yan, F., Cao, H., Chaturvedi, R., Krishna, U., Hobbs, S. S., Dempsey, P. J., & Polk, D. B. (2009). Epidermal growth factor receptor activation protects gastric epithelial cells from Helicobacter pylori-induced apoptosis. Gastroenterology, 136(4), 1297–1307.e3. https://doi.org/10.1053/j.gastro.2008.12.059.

150. Younes, M. (2013). Molecular pathology of Barrett's metaplasia and esophageal adenocarcinoma. In A. R. Sepulveda & J. P. Lynch (Eds.), Molecular Pathology of Neoplastic Gastrointestinal Diseases (pp. 43–52). Springer US. https://doi.org/10.1007/978-1-4614-6015-2_3.

151. Zhang, K., Chen, L., Zhu, C., Zhang, M., & Liang, C. (2023). Current knowledge of Th22 cell and IL-22 functions in infectious diseases. Pathogens, 12(2), 176. https://doi.org/10.3390/pathogens12020176.

INDEX

D

E

F

G